SURROGACY

—— DREAMS COME TRUE ——

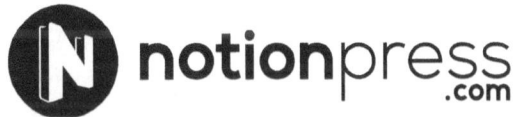

SURROGACY

—— DREAMS COME TRUE ——

An Experts View

DR. SANDEEP MANE

FRCOG (UK), CCST (UK), MD, DGO, FCPS, DICOG

Consultant in Reproductive Medicine and Surgery

Origin International Fertility Centre, Thane

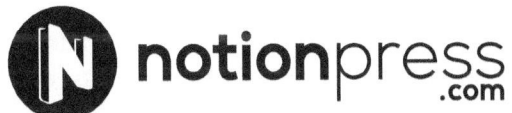

Notion Press

Old No. 38, New No. 6
McNichols Road, Chetpet
Chennai - 600 031

First Published by Notion Press 2017
Copyright © Dr. Sandeep Mane 2017
All Rights Reserved.

ISBN 978-1-946983-33-6

This book has been published with all reasonable efforts taken to make the material error-free after the consent of the author. No part of this book shall be used, reproduced in any manner whatsoever without written permission from the author, except in the case of brief quotations embodied in critical articles and reviews.

The Author of this book is solely responsible and liable for its content including but not limited to the views, representations, descriptions, statements, information, opinions and references ["Content"]. The Content of this book shall not constitute or be construed or deemed to reflect the opinion or expression of the Publisher or Editor. Neither the Publisher nor Editor endorse or approve the Content of this book or guarantee the reliability, accuracy or completeness of the Content published herein and do not make any representations or warranties of any kind, express or implied, including but not limited to the implied warranties of merchantability, fitness for a particular purpose. The Publisher and Editor shall not be liable whatsoever for any errors, omissions, whether such errors or omissions result from negligence, accident, or any other cause or claims for loss or damages of any kind, including without limitation, indirect or consequential loss or damage arising out of use, inability to use, or about the reliability, accuracy or sufficiency of the information contained in this book.

Dedication

This book is dedicated to my parents,
Mr Vishwas Mane and Mrs Vasanti Mane

My children Miss Shrutika Mane and Master Rushabh Mane

My brothers, Dr Rajan Mane, Mr Pravin Mane and their families

All intended parents and

All Surrogate mothers

Contents

Acknowledgements   *ix*

Chapter 1: Infertility – A Stigma in India – A Curse – Why?	1
Chapter 2: Infertility – Treatment Options	7
Chapter 3: Surrogacy – A Treatment Option	17
Chapter 4: Surrogacy – Currently Compensatory Altruistic Not Commercial	68
Chapter 5: Regulation for Surrogacy – 2005 to 2014	72
Chapter 6: The Surrogacy Bill 2016 – Treatment Becomes Crime	79
Chapter 7: Surrogacy is a treatment. Adoption is a choice	87
Chapter 8: The World is more Commercial than Altruistic	91
Chapter 9: Surrogacy – The Media and the Peoples Opinion	94
Chapter 10: Surrogacy Solution – Please Heal it Not Kill	102
Chapter 11: FAQs-All Questions Must be Answered	112

Glossary   *115*

Acknowledgements

The author wishes to acknowledge the help of his entire Origin team in completing this project. This includes Dr Snehal Dhobale Kohale, Surrogacy team headed by Ms Disha R, Embryology team headed by Mrs Sangeetha K, Nursing team headed by Sister Mansi Dhule. Each member of the team has played a vital role in helping the Intended Parents and the Surrogate Mothers to have a safe and enjoyable journey to parenthood.

Special thanks to all intended parents, Mr and Mrs Jaiswal and to all the Surrogate mothers for sharing their personal story and photos in the book.

I am extremely grateful to Swami Yogachittam Saraswati for his continuous guidance and inspiration.

Chapter 1

Infertility – A Stigma in India – A Curse – Why?

Infertility is on the rise worldwide. It is no longer a private hidden sorrow as it is seen glaringly due to its increased incidence. One out of five couples is childless and this number is constantly on the rise. In the cities, about 15% of the married women are childless. The rate of infertility is found higher in women with increasing levels of education. Working women are 20% more likely to be infertile compared to the Non-working women. This could be due to the priority given to the career, causing higher age at marriage, stress lifestyles, poor eating habits, etc

Chart 1: Reasons for Infertility

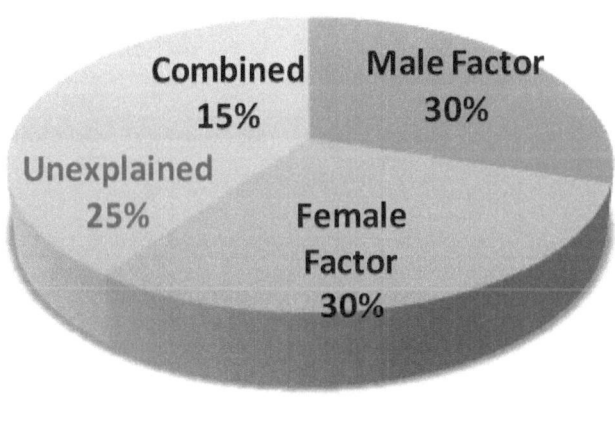

■ Male   ■ Female   ■ Combined   ■ Unexplainrd

The Reasons for Infertility Include: (Chart 1)

Male Infertility (due to sperm abnormalities in the man) – 30%.

10% of men have severe sperm abnormality. 90 million Indian men suffer from erectile dysfunction. This can happen due to genetic reasons, infections, injury to the testis, excessive heat, smoking and alcohol.

Female Infertility (Due to abnormalities of the egg, tubes or uterus) – 30%

The underlying causes include infections such as tuberculosis, pelvic infections, obesity, stress, pelvic surgery, ovarian failure, endometriosis and fibroids.

Combined (male and Female) – 15%

Unexplained (all tests appear to be normal, but there is difficulty in conception) – 25%

Chart 2: Implications of Infertility

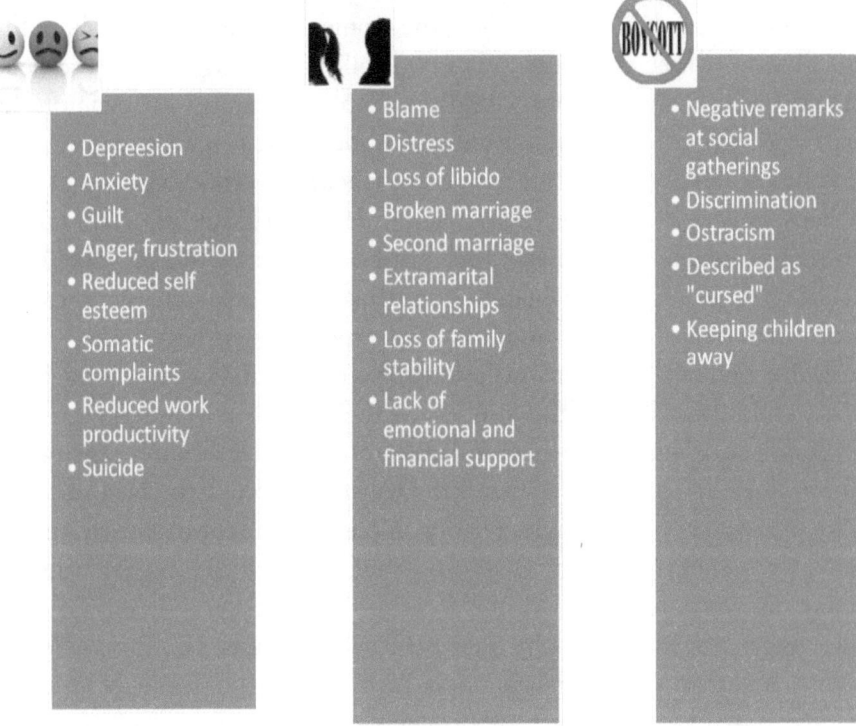

EMOTIONAL
- Depreesion
- Anxiety
- Guilt
- Anger, frustration
- Reduced self esteem
- Somatic complaints
- Reduced work productivity
- Suicide

MARITAL
- Blame
- Distress
- Loss of libido
- Broken marriage
- Second marriage
- Extramarital relationships
- Loss of family stability
- Lack of emotional and financial support

SOCIAL
- Negative remarks at social gatherings
- Discrimination
- Ostracism
- Described as "cursed"
- Keeping children away

In India, this is not just a medical problem, but a huge social issue for the couple. People in the west believe that India does not need fertility treatment centre's, because we are an overpopulated country. Indians wonder why infertile couples want babies with their own genes. The purpose of life is to experience the joy of childhood, youth, adulthood, parenthood and so on. Each individual desires to have this experience in life and it is a very personal matter, which has emotions and feelings attached to it.

The couple, irrespective of their caste, religion or nationality, faces personal, interpersonal, family, social and religious pressures at every moment of their life. In Hinduism, the women are expected to follow the stri dharma, which is to bear the responsibility of giving birth to the heirs of the family, especially sons. Childless people, voluntarily or involuntarily are faced with a form of isolation by the society. It is hard to understand the mindset behind this. Normal people (those who conceive simply) find it hard to accept that the couple facing delays in conception are just as normal as anyone else and that they just need some assistance. There is no justification in boycotting them from birthdays, weddings, christenings and family functions. In events and functions, even strangers have no hesitation in asking personal questions such as: Are you married, For How long, How many children and so on. This only makes their situation worse and it is hard to understand that this behavior come from even close family members. The women are generally assumed to be at fault, even if the husband may have the problem. The couples relationship is put under extreme strain and it is a real test of their ability to stay together. Amidst this constant pressure, internally and externally, with the emotional, physical and financial strain, the couple continues to fight their own battle **(Chart 2)**. Those who are able to maintain their marriage under such conditions, especially in India, are the most "made for each other" couples. It is sheer commitment and their love for each other, due to which they stay together under such strain. It is much easier for couples to stay together when they have children as a common reason for the relationship. The couple feels a sense of failure, isolation from the society, grief, loss, depression and suicidal even. At some stage, they lose their libido and they may even start the blame game, which is then fuelled by their families. These couples must be supported by their families, the society and the medical experts so that they can achieve their ultimate goal of life, to achieve a baby. Unfortunately, our culture demands that for the woman to be socially acceptable, she must have at least one biological child.

Family Pressures: The stigma even extends to their family members such as the siblings, in-laws, parents, who are highly disappointed by the inability of the couple to conceive. In some cases, the younger sibling may be under pressure to wait till the elder brother or sister can conceive. Occasionally, the younger sibling achieves a conception soon and this builds the pressure on the elder couple. This can all result in tremendous strain within the family. Some parents have even disowned their children, because they have been unable to conceive.

Emotional Strain: If the woman does not get the support from her husband, then she is in serious trouble, in the marriage, the family and the society. In such situations, the husband is under pressure to do a second marriage. She may be suffering from depression and emotional frustration resulting from the repeated treatment failures and regular visits to the doctors. She is likely to lose her libido and if the husband is not supportive, this can constitute grounds for divorce according to a recent court judgment. In India, 67% of women do not work, 80% have not been educated. How can one expect these women to stand up and fight. Lack of education and financial dependence makes them crippled and helpless.

Financial Strain: The National Family Health Survey found that women with low standard of living have high infertility compared to women with medium or high standards of living. Prolonged treatment leads to financial exhaustion along with emotional and physical strain. At the same time, there is a pressure to continue the treatment, because the age of the woman matters to the outcome of the treatment. She may be dependent and may not have much say in the financial matters. One has to imagine the plight of such a person. This is the reality of the woman suffering from infertility.

The couple may decide to come to terms with the situation and wish to stay alone, but the family, rituals and the society remain unwilling to accept their decision to stay childless. Due to this, the couple goes in cycles of treatment, withdrawl and treatment again. They have no idea when this will finish. It appears to them that life is about ultrasound scans, blood tests, hospital visits and a month after month battle starting with the onset of periods. In India, family and friends even keep a track of the woman's period dates. Inquisitive relatives have the audacity to ring and enquire each month. They enjoy gossiping, taunting and start giving free advise to the couple. The distraught couple is highly confused to be able to decide what is right or wrong. In no time, they have accumulated files of different doctors. The pile of files keep getting bigger, because they lose patience and trust if they do not get mental satisfaction with the treating doctor.

Effect of Infertility on the Couple: Marriage without children is considered as a failure of the two individuals. The couple prefers to stay isolated as this becomes the topic of discussion in every family or social event they attend. They start getting a feeling of guilt, shame and even low self esteem. The lack of respect shown by the near and dear ones becomes tough to handle. These couples are under tremendous pressure to prove to themselves, their family and the society that they are as normal as the others. Just like a person with some disability is considered Not normal, similarly, an infertile couple especially a woman and that too in India has a lot to prove. It becomes harder and harder for the couple to believe that sooner or later they will overcome the problem and have a baby. They start feeling hopeless, but most of them pretend to be fine. The couples may start feeling that they are a burden on the society.

Chapter 2
Infertility – Treatment Options

Young couples enter into a relationship and start to explore the ways ahead. In the Indian culture, sex is a taboo and is hardly discussed openly in any family. There is an element of negativity attached to it, especially in women. This can have a detrimental effect in the new couples life. For some couples, the struggles start at that stage. There is so much on the minds of a newly wed bride when she goes to stay with the husbands family at the in-laws house. Apart from handling the emotional turmoil of leaving her parents home, she is faced with a new start of numerous other relations. She has to adjust to her husbands ways. She may or may not be working. This may add a completely new dimension to the new couples life at the in-laws house. After all this, they have to start their married life. It is very common that physical relations may not happen well. This is an issue that they cannot discuss openly in the family and friends. Hence, they get very little proper advise which can help them. They suffer in silence. In some cases, the jobs may be demanding or the husband and wife may do a lot of travelling and may not be able to spend enough time together to be able to conceive. If all is well, the couple may have planned their life and might want to deliberately delay their conception. This may not be acceptable to the family and pressure may start to build on the couple. The brunt of the anger is taken by the woman. The Indian tradition of considering periods to be unholy makes it easy for everyone around her to know that she is having her periods. Even if she wishes to keep it to herself, she has to unfortunately declare to the whole world that even this month has not been successful. This may even lead to a family discussion on the subject and the politics may start amongst the various family members.

If a couple has tried to conceive by regular natural relations for a duration of about 2 years, conception is expected to happen. If not, the worries start at this stage. Numerous advises are given to visit the doctors and the couple gets inundated with recommendations. Finally, they choose to visit a doctor. They find it embarrassing to enter a fertility clinic, because the purpose of visit becomes obvious. Amidst this, when they meet the doctor, their anxiety levels would shoot up. They would hope that they would be sorted by simple advise of some tablets **(Chart 3)**. This is when their personal life is explored by the doctor. No one would like this, but they have no choice but to share this information. If they are in the right place, this discussion may be gentle and they may walk out feeling good. On the other hand, if they are treated like a vegetable, then their pains have just started. This journey could involve 5, 10, 15 , 20 or 30 years visits to the doctors.

Chart 3: Stepwise Approach to Treatment of Infertility

- Natural relations — 1 to 2 years
- Determine the cause
- Ovulation tabs + Natural — 4 months
- Ovulation tabs + Natural + IUI — 4 months

  About 3 years from marriage

- Role of Laparoscopy and Hysteroscopy
  Ovulation tabs/Inj + Natural + IUI — 3 to 4 months

  About 5 years from marriage

- IVF / ICSI
- The above plan may change as per the woman's age and other factors

Treatment options for Infertility & Success Rate

Sr No	Treatment	Success Rate
1	Ovulation Tablets + Natural	3 to 5 %
2	Ovulation Tablets/Injections + IUI	15 to 20 %
3	IVF/ICSI	50 to 60 %

The next thing that the couple has to do is the medical reports. The wife has to do blood tests and the unpleasant internal sonography. The husband undergoes blood tests and is asked to collect semen sample in toilets in most places. This marks the beginning of the couples agony. In some cases, this becomes the routine of their lives for many more years to come. The only difference is that it may happen at different clinics and at different intervals with different doctors.

Once the test reports are available, the couple visits the doctors to understand the reports and take suggestions for their treatment. This can be a very nervous moment for the couple. Doctors who do this 15 times a day may forget that this is the first time for this couple in their life. They are unaware of the future implications and are now very scared. They want reassurance, hope and a comfort feeling that the doctor will help them without making it very difficult for them. This is where standardization of care would matter. The communication skills and the doctors ability to reassure the couple would make a big difference. The reports are informed to the couple and the underlying cause may be found. As seen in the chart, the treatment start with simple natural cycles that may be aided with tablets for egg formation to be given for just 5 days. The worst part is that doctors start advising the couple to maintain natural relations on certain days of the woman's menstrual cycle. This leads the couple to look at the calendar and mark the days to keep relations, irrespective of whether they feel like or not. Now the natural act has become a treatment for this couple. Like taking pills, relations are also kind of prescribed. The natural act becomes a mechanical event for the sperms to be deposited in the right place with a hope that the test comes positive. Imagine the tension on the couple at the end of the month heading towards the day of the period to see if the pregnancy test comes positive. In the meantime, if the woman starts getting symptoms of period, she has already started going into depression. From now on, this may happen every month end for years to come. It is not surprising that the couple loses interest in relations, because the natural act is based on emotional satisfaction and not for just baby making.

As this starts happening, the couple starts planning their work commitments around the days of their treatment. The number of leaves start going up. The performance at work drops. This is even more in the case of the woman who needs to take more time off from work. In the process, some women take the disastrous decision of resigning from work. This now means that every moment of their life is about the period dates, sonographies, injections, timed relations and pregnancy test. How long can one tolerate this. The relation start getting the dents. The happiness of marriage and the excitement of wanting a family have disappeared in thin air. The couple starts to have excessive sex, they go on holidays and try to bury their emotions. When this approach does not work, the couple is now getting impatient and finally anger sets in. They get disappointed by their own bodies, their families, doctors and even god.

This leads the family machinery to come into play. Visits to temples, Babaji's, fasts at regular intervals, pujas, and all ways to bring good fortune are tried. The couple starts to feel that science may not be just enough. Any rational person also may start becoming superstitious under these circumstances. It is hard to convince them to avoid such actions, because the family pressures are now very high on them.

A pregnancy test may suddenly come positive at some stage and then it could be in the tube, an en ectopic pregnancy, which has to be removed as it is dangerous. If it is in the womb, the couple waits anxiously for 3 weeks to perform the first sonography. This may not show a heartbeat and the couples excitement crashes. They go blank and are unable to understand anything that is being explained to them. The woman may undergo the curetting procedure to clear the unhealthy remains of the pregnancy. This becomes emotionally challenging for the couple, because all their hopes have just got shattered and they now have to restart the whole process again. Some women go into depression. The men also suffer silently. They have to continue their jobs and have to keep earning to be able run their home and also to fund further treatment. At some stage, the couple must be feeling that they are earning only to spend on their medical treatment.

If the simple approach does not work, the couple is advised to take the next step, which is normally IUI (Intrauterine insemination). This involves taking the tablets again for 5 days, followed by regular scans to check the growth of the egg. When the egg is ready as per the scan, an injection is given to release it at a fixed time. At this time, the husband gives a semen sample. This is then processed to select the best sperms to put in the right place (womb) at the right time (egg release time) by a fine catheter. This has a nominal success rate of 15 to 17%. This means that the chances of failure are very high and the treatment has to be done repeatedly sometimes.

If this is not working, the couple may lose their faith in the doctor and go to another clinic. Unfortunately, the tests may have become old and the doctors may wish to repeat the tests. Now this clinic may have its own different arrangements. The couple is now dealing with new staff and doctors and that must be challenging. Sometimes, couples travel a long distance to undergo the treatment from a particular clinic and this can have a serious impact on their sufferings.

If three to four IUIs do not work, the couple is getting fedup and may take a break to relax a little. If they are not counseled properly at this stage, they may keep doing too many IUIs. In the process, they start taking excessive medications, which can harm them later and reduce the chances of success using the advanced treatment. This must be avoided at all costs. It is very important that the couple understands the full process and is doing the treatment with complete knowledge.

When they are ready to restart their treatment, they are now faced with some difficult choices. The first is to consider one or two more IUIs to keep the treatment simple and the second is to perform a laparoscopy and hysteroscopy and then some more IUIs. Laparoscopy and Hysteroscopy is an operation involving small cuts on the woman's tummy. A fine telescope is introduced inside the tummy to check if the tubes are open and if there are any other undetected issues. If any problem, such as a tubal block, fibroid or endometriosis is found, it should be treated at the same sitting. In some centre's, such facilities and skills may not exist for the operative part and that part is performed at a later date again. This leads to doubling of the effort and should be avoided preferably. In some women, this operation gets performed repeatedly and leads to increased pain, sufferings and costs.

In the process of trying tablets, IUIs and maybe laparoscopy and hysteroscopy, most of the times two more years have gone by. The couple may be about 5 years into the marriage. The age of the woman and the family pressures are increasing. They are fedup and tired of doing the IUIs and follicular sonographies. This may appear to be a simple form of the treatment, but it starts appearing to be meaningless. They are now getting mentally ready to move further into the advanced form of the treatment (IVF-test-tube baby). They start to gather the information and then visit the doctor to understand the treatment and its costs. At this stage, the couple has started to wonder if the medications are going to have any side effects on the woman. Once they are reassured, they are now willing to do the test-tube baby treatment sooner or later. Some couples have to discuss this at home and convince them to agree for this treatment.

Sometimes, the parents and in-laws may discuss the cost burden to be shared. If the understanding is low, the friction can start at this stage.

The couple prepares their funds, makes arrangements at home for help during the treatment, organizes leave and take a leap into the treatment. They are well aware that this treatment is now appearing to be necessary even though they dislike this choice. It is no more a matter of like or dislike. The worst part of this treatment is that it spans over a period of almost a month and involves almost daily injections and regular blood tests and sonographies. On top, there is no guarantee of success. This is perceived by many as the business of the fertility industry. It is sad that many who do not understand a thing about the couples tragedy and about the science of this treatment make such allegations on doctors who are making every effort over prolonged periods to get a success for the couple. The treatment needs a good facility, technology, costly medications and skilled staff, which costs a lot. None of this comes cheap. Each fertility clinic has its own arrangements, but if this is not up to the mark, the couple can have a horrible experience. Once the eggs are collected from the lady, they are mixed with the sperms in the laboratory under very sterile culture conditions. This results in the formation of the embryos (early pregnancy). The good embryos are the selected and transferred to the womb for the pregnancy to implant (stick) and grow for nine months. Unfortunately, at this stage, nature takes over and it can fail. If it comes positive, it is hard for them to believe it at first. This is just the start of another opportunity to have a baby. Unfortunately, the pregnancy can again be in the tube (ectopic) or may miscarry. If all goes well, they are now in a dilemma whether to disclose the information to family and friends. They are afraid that if anything goes wrong in the pregnancy after disclosing to the world, it would be very difficult to handle the situation.

Failed first IVF attempt: If the result comes negative, it is a tragedy for the couple. The failure of the first IVF cycle is one of the most difficult moments in the entire treatment of this couple. The first experience feels very intensive as it is all very new for the couple. There is a lot to take in and lot to cope with on the personal front. Even at this stage, they are hoping for a miraculous natural pregnancy. When this first attempt of IVF treatment fails, the couple realizes that the issue is slightly more serious than they thought. Their minds open to undergo further treatment, because this looks like the only way forward. The failure of the first attempt is analyzed and the couple is given a feedback about the performance of the cycle and the details regarding the eggs, sperms and the uterus. On this basis, the couple understands the reason for the failure, the available treatment options and then they decide about the timing of their next treatment. By this time, most couples are clearly rattled by the situation and get mentally disturbed. They may take time to settle and then restart the process. If the experience with the first clinic is unpleasant, the couple is likely to change the doctor. In this case, some tests get repeated and a fresh attempt is then undertaken.

How Many Attempts of IVF? (Chart 4)

It is believed that IVF treatment should be successful atleast by the third attempt. If pregnancy does not happen after three attempts, it is obvious that the nature capacity is not looking favorable. The egg, sperm or the uterus could be responsible for the failure, but it is the egg, which is most likely. A change of eggs may become necessary in some cases. This can be a very emotional consultation and each couple responds very differently to this situation. The first feeling is that of denial and disbelief, followed by anger and then acceptance. The couple may get angry on themselves for some of the decisions that may have gone wrong. They may have delayed the treatment due to which natural body changes may have started. This phase of transition from self eggs to donor eggs can be of 2 minutes in some cases, few months in some and never in some rare cases. It is a very personal call and it is not about right or wrong. It is about the preparation of the mind to accept borrowed eggs or sperms. The pregnancy will be carried by the wife and no one will know about the change of the eggs or sperms.

Chart 4: Advanced Treatment options for Infertility-IVF & Success Rate

	Egg	Sperm	Uterus	Success Rate
Option 1	Own	Own	Own	30 to 40 %
Option 2	Donor	Own	Own	50 to 60 %
Option 3	Own	Donor	Own	50 to 60 %
Option 4	Donor	Donor	Own	50 to 60 %
Option 5	Own	Own	Surrogate	60 to 70 %
Option 6	Donor	Own	Surrogate	70 to 80 %
Option 7	Adoption			

Reproduction is an important natural instinct and it is equally important for people to have their own genes. It is insensitive to advise someone to adopt against their own wish when they can have a child using their own eggs and sperms. It takes a lot of mental preparation for anyone to have a child without their own eggs and sperms. It is very personal and individuals respond to this decision very differently. For a small number of people, this is a very easy decision. A small number would never go ahead, because they would rather remain childless. In majority of the people, their mind agrees to use borrowed eggs and sperms (if medically required), but only after they understand the medical situation and when they are thoroughly counseled about the options available to them. Borrowing of eggs, sperms from a donor or the more advanced options such as surrogacy and adoption are generally undertaken as last options by any couple. As no treatment option guarantees an outcome, it is important to be systematic and progressive in the treatment. Every effort is made by the couple and their doctors to achieve conception quickly and by using their own eggs and sperms in their own womb. If for any reason this is not possible, then they get ready for the next level of treatment. In the process, it gets tougher and tougher for them, because the decisions are getting harder and the costs are rising. The risks of failure are still looming on their head. They have only three options, stop and wait for a miracle to happen, make further attempts or to adopt.

At all times, the above options are explained to the couple. It is a choice they make on the basis of their personal feelings, circumstances and their risk taking capability. Most couples get successful and this is a unique moment for the couple as well as their treating doctors. Every effort is made by the medical team to achieve success. It is unfortunate that some poor practices bring bad name to the entire fraternity. Regulations will go a long way in achieving higher standards of care and the patients and the other involved parties will all get just and fair treatment.

Repeated IVF Treatment Failures

In most cases, a pregnancy is achieved during the first three IVF attempts, either using the couples own eggs or borrowed eggs. The multiple attempts take a huge toll on the couples capacity to continue further-emotionally, physically and financially. By this time, the couple could be in the marriage for anything between 7 to 20 years. The husband and wife have reached an advanced age and they start felling hopeless. They are faced with difficult decisions about the path ahead almost daily. The temptation to continue never finishes. They still keep hoping that they can have a pregnancy using their own eggs and sperms. Even if they have decided to borrow eggs, they would still like the pregnancy in themselves. The thought of surrogacy is still difficult to accept. Some of them gradually start thinking of the options ahead for them. They meet the doctors, surf the internet and try to find out about surrogacy and even adoption. Even though the couple has undergone numerous years of fertility treatment, they have never understood the way surrogacy works.

To Stop the Treatment, do Surrogacy or to Adopt

When the treatment goes to the final stage, the couple is faced with three options-To stop the treatment, Surrogacy or Adoption. This decision is influenced by three factors:

a) Their personal feelings

b) The family view

c) The social acceptance

The couple is open to all options, but they fear the risk of failing and most importantly, the social acceptance. India is still ingrained with cultural beliefs and a conservative thought process. The society is unwilling to accept childless couples, surrogate children and adoption. The couple prefers to do something rather than stay childless. This means it comes down to Surrogacy or Adoption.

The Role of the Medical Experts

In India, the fertility treatment available to patients in various cities and clinics is not always standardized. The strategy mentioned above is theoretically understood, but the practical implementation is challenging. This has numerous reasons such as lack of proper training to doctors in some cases, lack of facilities in some private clinics, lack of skills of the sonologists, endoscopic surgeons and embryologist. Communication skills is still an underdeveloped area in the medical practice in India. Postgraduate training from government medical colleges does not allow enough scope for doctors to sharpen their communication skills. Counseling is the most important aspect of fertility treatment. Doctors need to be able to give adequate time for patients to understand the issues. It is vital that the patients understand the reasons for their delay in conception and the way forward for them. Mental preparation and education of the couple is the cornerstone of successful fertility treatment. Patience and Trust are needed in abundance and this is only possible if the patients feel confident in the doctor and the clinic. Patients are willing to travel to far distances in search of a good facility. They want a personal touch during their treatment.

If the strategy goes wrong, it has a disastrous effect on the future treatment of the patient. A lot of valuable time, money and energy may be lost unnecessarily.

Chapter 3

Surrogacy – A Treatment Option

What is Surrogacy?

Surrogacy is when another woman carries and gives birth to a baby for a couple who is desiring to have a child and is unable to do so themselves.

History of Surrogacy

In 1978, the first test-tube baby (IVF baby), Louise Brown, was born in England. Soon after, in 1980, Noel Keane made the first official legal surrogacy agreement. In 1985, the first surrogate mother carried a successful pregnancy. Conservative estimates show that more than 25,000 children are now being born through surrogates in India every year.

Intended Parents – Their Journey Towards Surrogacy?

Al most all couples who come to this stage of treatment have been through years of fertility treatment and have been unsuccessful to have their own child. In this process, they become emotionally, physically and financially weak and are unable to keep their efforts going. They become hopeless and are unable to continue further. During these years of trying they suffer as a couple, they suffer from the family pressures and disappointments, they suffer due to the societal torture and they also suffer in their professional career leading to financial difficulties. Their whole life is revolving around this one thing- to have a baby. This is so easily possible for the majority of the people that they are unable to appreciate the difficulty faced by the infertile couple. The couples going for surrogacy have finished their patience. Most of them are depressed and some even suicidal. Life appears meaningless to them. Every day they have to make an effort to raise their spirits and find ways to keep themselves occupied.

After all the initial efforts of simple treatment, they are now left with the following options:

a) Stop all treatment and just give up: This is a very difficult option and is almost impossible to live like this, because the family and society will constantly remind this couple of their infertility.

b) Continue the same treatment that has been unsuccessful for years and is looking hopeless. This leads to even worse physical and mental agony and all the money and energy gets wasted even further.

c) Take the help of another woman who is willing to help them to carry and a deliver a baby for them. This option becomes their preferred choice, because this has a high success rate. On a personal front, the couple gets mentally ready to accept this option due to the huge suffering of the prolonged treatment, which makes them feel hopeless. The couple needs to be mentally ready to accept this. Then they start wondering if their families will accept surrogacy and finally, they think about their strategy to handle the society. Very few people understand this option of surrogacy. It is ignorance due to which loose comments are made and the couple is discouraged. The husband and wife would both like their genes in the baby. This is a natural instinct, which continues to be their first choice all throughout. In most cases, the treatment has consumed a lot of time and the wife's age is advanced by the time they get to surrogacy. Before they even think of surrogacy, the couple is likely to have tried their own treatment using donor (borrowed) eggs. These are the reasons for the couple to accept donor eggs and surrogacy in some cases. It can be possible to have a baby with eggs and sperms of the desiring couple in the surrogate mother. It is absolutely mandatory that at least the eggs or the sperms belong to the couple. Surrogacy cannot be done if there is no genetic link to the desiring couple. When the couple is educated about this option, in today's situation, couples are willing to take this option.

Surrogacy Done in Unusual Situations

Absence of uterus from birth

Developmental abnormalities of the womb can happen in any woman **(Chart 5)**. This happens at the time of the formation of the body and can be of different types such as- a very small size, one half developed only, split into two halves and totally absent. These women are healthy and normal like anyone else till they come to puberty. They do not get their periods or get light periods and later on when they try for a baby, the diagnosis gets confirmed on a sonography.

Chart 5: Indications for Surrogacy

Uterine Problems
- Absent Uterus
- Hypoplstic Uterus
- Hysterectomy (Uterus removal)

Medical Conditions
(Making Pregnancy Risky)
- Heart disease, Kidney disease, Severe Hypertension, Connective tissue disorders etc

Other Reasons
- Recurrent miscarriage
- Recurrent IVF failures
- Advanced maternal age

Serious health conditions in the woman

Creating risk to life if she becomes pregnant. Some women suffer from serious health disorders such as heart disease, kidney disease, bleeding disorders and many such conditions in which carrying a pregnancy and delivery poses a risk of death to the woman and also the baby. These conditions may be known to them from an early age. If they get married, there may be an understanding with the husband about the condition and they may want o have a baby using surrogacy.

Single Parents

Single men may desire to have a pregnancy. This matter has raised some questions about surrogacy. This is not a medical matter for the doctors to decide the correctness of this indication for surrogacy. This is a social and constitutional matter and needs a legal guidance. This should be decided on the grounds of human and constitutional grounds. This is a rare request and should not question the legitimacy of the entire treatment. Carefully designed fair eligibility criteria can easily take care of this matter.

Same Sex Couples, Especially Gay Men

This is also a social and constitutional matter. Legal guidance will help us decide if this should be done or not. There are changing times and it is for the honorable courts to advise the medical experts about what they are allowed to do.

Divorced Individuals, Especially with Children from their Past Relationship

It is unfair to assume that divorced individuals cannot be good parents. Disallowing them to do surrogacy appears to infringe on their human rights. In this case also, the honorable courts can decide their eligibility.

Surrogacy for NRIs and OCI Card Holders

It is hard to understand that we wish to discriminate against the NRIs and OCIs on the grounds that they have higher divorce rates. Most of these Indians have stayed abroad for some years and are passionate about their country. For some personal reasons, they may be staying abroad. There are many who are returning to India for good. Our Prime Minister has been urging them to return to India and invest in our country. It will be fair to allow them to undertake surrogacy. Very few will actually need this treatment, but it will send a positive message to all the others who feel so strongly for their country. The gesture will help to build confidence in this group of Indians.

Surrogacy for Foreign Nationals

Medical services should not be limited by boundaries such as caste, religion or nationality. If stringent rules are made, then this can be done within the given framework. The unborn child should not be at risk of being stateless. This can be ensured by a written confirmation from the embassy to which the couple belongs. This was already being done at the time when ban for implemented. The problem relating to foreigners had almost finished after the new rules and regulations as per the ICMR guidelines were followed.

Surrogacy by Couples who Already have their Own Children

This is to be decided by the honorable courts of this country on the basis of human rights issue. It is a constitutional decision and not medical at all.

Surrogacy - Dreams Come True

Chart 6a: Life Journey of Intended Parents and Surrogate Mothers

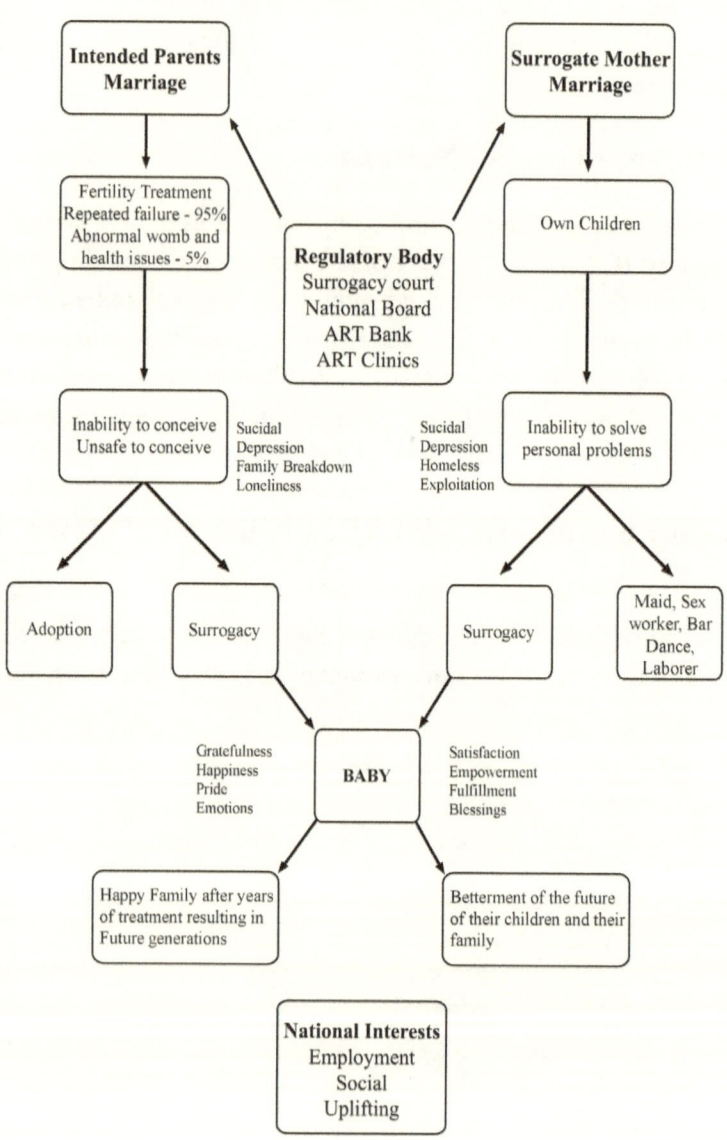

Surrogate Mothers – Their Journey Towards Surrogacy

The story of the surrogate mothers: India has a large number of people living in poverty and an equally large number of lower middle class people who need more and more money for basic needs such as good shelter, education for children and an improvement in the living standard. The women in this group are mostly uneducated and unskilled. They have been brought up with the idea of living at their husbands home, produce children and do their upbringing. Most of them have never ventured out of their homes in search of jobs to make an earning. These women suddenly face the harsh reality of life. Their husband may die, disappear or dump the woman with her children. Sometimes, husbands may abandon their wives with the children, just because they have lost interest in them or because they only have daughters. Leaving their wives due to infertility in them is another reason why women find themselves helpless in the middle of their young lives. Natural calamities such as famine and floods are a common occurrence in India **Chart 6**. They may wish to upgrade their houses or give better education to their children. They may get robbed or cheated and cannot manage the finances. They may be farmers and are in debt. Every day is a new struggle to survive, let alone education and the luxuries of life.

What Makes them Choose Surrogacy?

Young women coming for surrogacy may or may not be with their husbands, but they certainly lack education, skills and any form of capability to do a good employment. They are young, decent, brave and determined. They want to survive and do something for their children and the family. They speak to their neighbors and friends to explore the options available to them. Some may suggest to do household maid work, cook or work at construction site. Nowadays, even this is not easy, because employers want references. They become very vulnerable. These desperate helpless women become very unsafe. Some may get sexually exploited. Financial exploitation is almost guaranteed. They have no one to protect them. Some find the wrong company who guide them towards bar dancing and sex working. It is hard to understand which option is best for them. When we talk of employment for surrogate mothers, which one mentioned in **Chart 7** is being suggested. Which option protects them from exploitation, in fact, they will face a lot more exploitation if they are left to their own fate.

Chart 7: Options Available to the Surrogate Mother

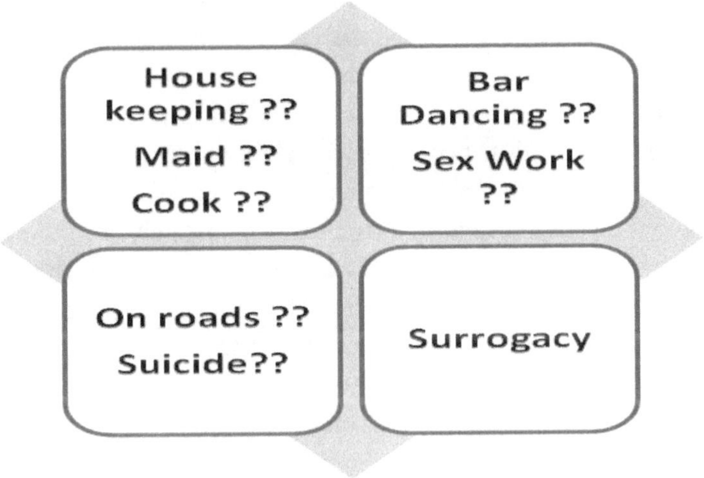

House keeping ?? Maid ?? Cook ??	Bar Dancing ?? Sex Work ??
On roads ?? Suicide??	Surrogacy

By doing surrogacy, the woman is able to educate her children or save some for the difficult days ahead.

Surrogacy: Bringing Happiness (Chart 6b)

Types of Surrogacy

There are two types of surrogacy:

1. Altruistic Surrogacy
2. Commercial Surrogacy

Altruistic Surrogacy

Altruism means selflessness and it is the opposite of selfishness **(Chart 8)**. In simple terms, altruism means caring about the welfare of other people with the objective of helping them. Does this make a surrogate mother totally selfish just because she has been compensated for helping someone. The amount paid is compensatory in nature and not commercial. She is doing it with intentions of caring for her children, her family and the intended parents. Just because she is giving away the child at the end of the nine months, does she become a emotionless machine. These are responsible individuals remaining true to their word given in the contract. She may be in control of her emotions, but that does not make her inhuman and selfish. Is it really possible that they do not care for the baby and that only the money matters to them. Can this be the conclusion of their big-heartedness. The birth of a baby is not an isolated event, it is the birth of generations for that family. What amount of money will qualify for this to be called a commercial business. The current form of surrogacy is Altruistic, compensatory at the most, if we calculate the magnitude of the outcome.

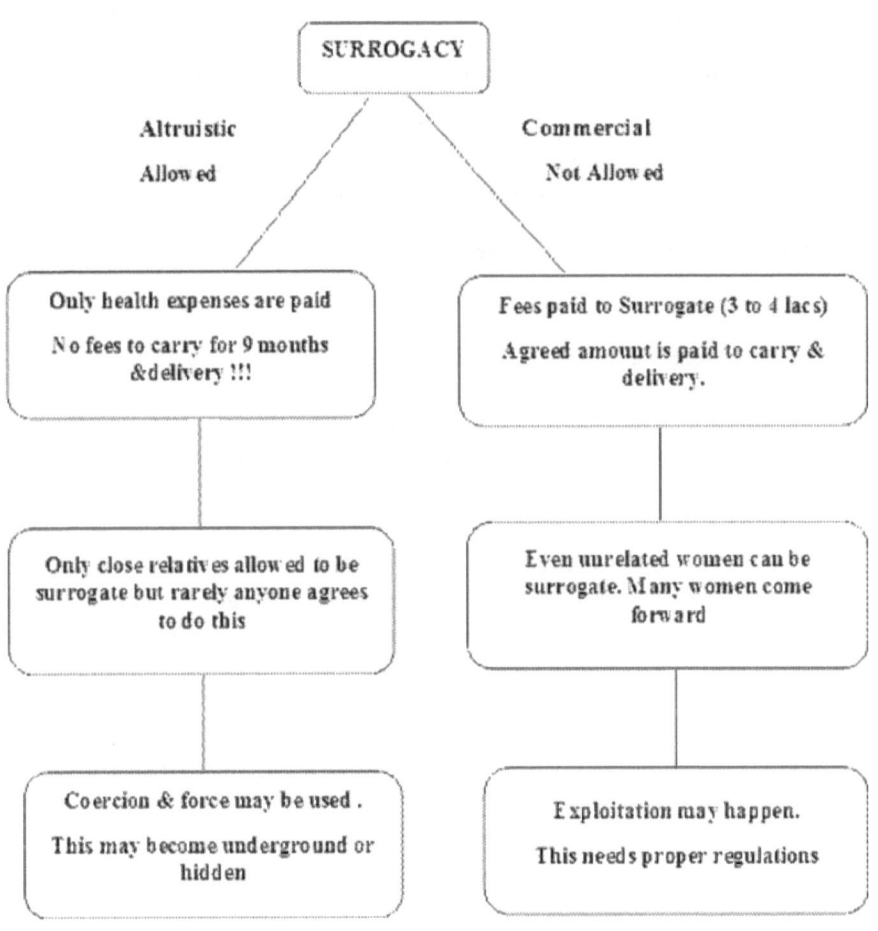

Chart 8: Altruistic and Commercial Surrogacy

In altruistic surrogacy, patients will only be allowed to pay medical bills of the surrogate mothers and no other payments can be made. The logic is that if any amount is paid, it becomes commercial in nature. This concept raises a lot of questions for other similar situations.

Should the doctor even charge fees for using his intelligence

Should the coolie on the station charge for using his muscles to lift your bags

Should labourers on the construction sites and the municipal cleaners charge

Using your body to earn money-brain or hand or eyes or muscles- why not stop taking anything in return for this

Musicians charge for their talent

Singers charge fees for their voice

Dancers use their bodies to charge fees

Cricketers earn handsome money by using their physical bodies

You pay to watch a circus where acrobatics are done

Altruism should not consider relationships. Is it not selfish if a close relative is helping the couple. It is for the benefit of the family in a selfish manner. True altruism is when you do the sacrifice for an unknown person. Does this happen in this day and age. The debate exists if true altruism is ever possible. In the act of helping, sharing and sacrificing without any exchange of money even, there is a selfishness involved. This is of a different form- personal gratification, spiritual well being, acquiring "punya" with rewards attached to it. These rewards could eventually take a monetary shape, intentionally or unintentionally.

Altruistic surrogacy is allowed in many countries but has not been proven to be a successful model. Example in countries like Australia, UK and Canada only altruistic surrogacy is allowed. When India allowed commercial surrogacy for foreign nationals, citizens of these countries flocked to India. The option of altruistic surrogacy was available in their country, but it was not viable for them.

Can the World Work on Altruism Alone???
Commercial Surrogacy

Commercial surrogacy was legalized in India in 2002 and has since grown to mammoth proportions since then. A World Bank study estimated the monetary value of surrogacy to be almost $2 billion, with 3,000 fertility clinics across India. The legal issues with commercial surrogacy surfaced when a couple from Japan divorced before the birth of their surrogate child. It exposed the Indian Law on Surrogacy to questions that had no clear answers.

Compensatory Not Commercial- Alternative Name to Surrogacy

The current form of surrogacy in India should be considered altruistic in nature, even with the compensatory nature of the treatment **Chart 9.** Altruism should be about good intentions even if it has a compensatory nature. The ultimate intentions in surrogacy is to relieve the pain and suffering of the intended parents by giving care to their baby and in the process she is helping her own children and family, There are reasons other than just financial gains that drive women to become surrogate mothers. Often, this reason is for the surrogate mothers to experience self-respect, empowerment and a sense of achievement and fulfillment of her responsibility towards her children and her family. There life gets a purpose with the blessings of a childless couple. They will carry the memories of giving the joy of parenthood to a helpless couple for the rest of their lives. The pride, blessings and joy will lift their spirits and lead to benefit for their children.

It is a sacrifice of the highest order. It deserves respect not shame. It is the biggest gift of life. It is the emotional, physical and divine gift from one human being to another.

The term commercial must be banned and instead "COMPENSATORY" should be used. The terms such as "Rent a womb," "Baby farms" and so on are coined by most westerners who are insulting motherhood. The parents and the surrogate mothers are good human beings helping each other to enjoy the experience of life. This process needs regulations so that the miscreants can be controlled and the treatment gets its deserved status of "PRIDE" and "RESPECT"

Surrogate mothers should be fairly compensated for the following reasons:

1) The time duration of almost one year that she donates
2) Loss of earnings- During the time of surrogacy, she is unable to work and this can have a compounding effect on her losses for her lifetime
3) She may need to employ help at home for looking after her children and her family
4) She loses valuable time that she could have spent with her family.
5) She makes a special effort during the pregnancy to ensure that all goes well.
6) Her health bills and her post-pregnancy care should be compensated

These heads can be objectively and practically evaluated and a fair compensation can be pre-determined. This can be controlled by the government through the national board so that the rules and regulations are followed. This must not have an exploitative nature, because the interests of the intended parents must also be safeguarded. The ultimate aim would be to bring fairness to all involved and stop any form of exploitation.

Chart 9: Compensatory Altruistic Surrogacy: Fee Structure

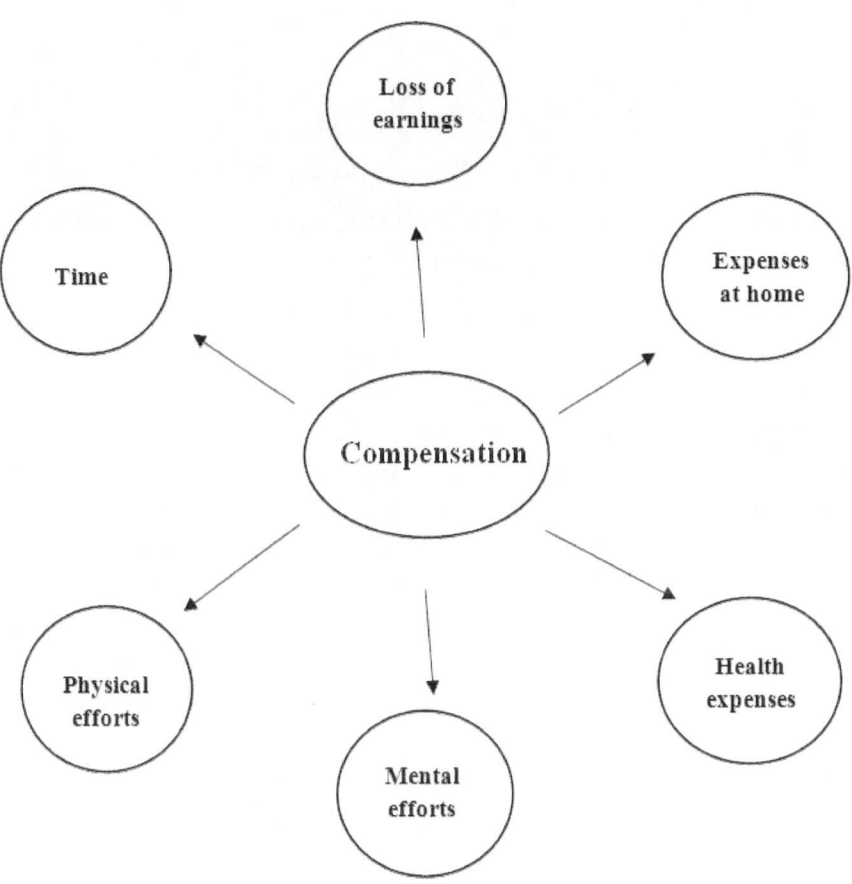

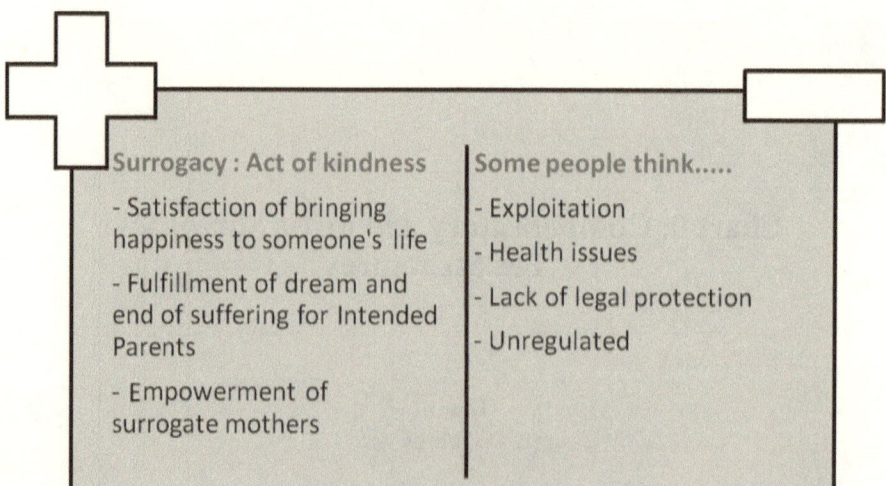

Medical Tourism: India Should be Proud to be the Number ONE Destination for Healthcare

Going abroad to the UK and USA for medical treatment was a fashion of the rich patients until recently. In a short span of last 10 years, our doctors have made us proud by making us the number 1 medical tourism industry in the world. The changing face of the country and the development of infrastructure, made us the 3rd best country in the world in terms of the quality of medical facilities and the services provided to patients. It is a nice feeling to be recognized and appreciated for good work than to be criticized as a most polluted, hungry country or a unhappy country and so on. The two Olympic medals (one silver and one bronze) won by the young Indian girls was a proud moment for the country. This is because, they got recognition for the quality of their game. Then, why is there a lack of enthusiasm in appreciating our medical fraternity for achieving the number one position in the world. The change in India is seen everywhere, but we are still not geared up to grab the opportunity that is lying ahead of us. These are changing times and India should learn to stand in pride and make its own decisions that are suitable for the country and its people. There should be no boundaries to offer medical treatment. All human beings are made by nature and we all live with a purpose of enjoying the experience of life. A doctor's job is to make a best effort to give the best experience to everyone. A doctor should not be offering treatment on the basis of caste, religion, nationality and so on. The governments should also not force doctors to discriminate between patients. Any patient from anywhere in the world, must be given healthcare in India at a fair cost. The governments must encourage this idea by regulating the process and safeguarding the patients, the doctors and the hospitals. We can lead the world by an example.

When do International Couples Travel Abroad for Treatment?

International couples decide to travel abroad at the stage when IVF attempts fail repeatedly. Couples travel to India from Africa, Europe, USA and many other countries. Generally, foreign couples tend to do their regular IVF treatments locally, but when there is repeated failure, they travel abroad for treatment. Most of these couples are of Indian Origin looking to undergo IVF treatment with own eggs or borrowed eggs. There are growing number of foreign couples who are coming to India for the advanced form of the treatment.

Benefits for the State are as Follows

- Working in the interests of its citizen
- Creation of new employment which will give benefit to the society
- Advancement in the field of fertility care on the global front
- Growth in tourism and travel

A well controlled, state-regulated surrogacy program will primarily benefit the surrogate mothers, the intended parents and also the nation. Prohibiting surrogacy for the international patients has declined the Medical Tourism in India which was at its peak in recent times.

Intended Parents- Their Stories and Opinions
Case 1: PK Story

Wifes age	:	**41 years**
Husbands age	:	**43 years**
Marriage	:	**15 years**
Reason for Surrogacy Treatment	:	**Severe health disorder with risk to life**

In September 2015, 41 year old wife with her 43 year old husband visited hospital with 15 years of married life & history of prior two miscarriages. Her prior two pregnancies had to be terminated at 4 month due to her medical condition. She was suffering from lupus nephritis, Idiopathic thrombocytopenic purpose & deep vein thrombosis, for which she was on immunosuppressive therapy & anticoagulant therapy. These are serious health conditions that can be life-threatening to the mother as well as risky for the pregnancy. Due to her medical condition & medications like warfarin it was not possible for her to carry pregnancy. So decision of donor egg – surrogacy was taken. Surrogate mother had positive result in first attempt. After uneventful 9 months, she delivered healthy baby girl.

Dr. Sandeep Mane

Case 1: PK Survey

1. Should Commercial Surrogacy Treatment be banned? Yes / **No**
2. Why did you choose to do Surrogacy? Fashion OR Treatment? Yes / **No**
3. Every person should have the right to choose the mode for their reproduction? **Agree** / Disagree
4. Genetic link to the child is important for every human being **Agree** / Disagree
5. Adoption cannot be forced on couples. **Agree** / Disagree
6. Could a close relative of yours have done Surrogacy for you? Yes / **No**
7. How should the surrogate mother feel after carrying a baby for you? **Proud** / Ashamed
8. Why you did not adopt a Child?
   We wanted to have _genetic link to the child._
9. Please tell us about your life before and after Surrogacy.
   A big void was filled in our life with joy and happiness.
10. What is your message to the government about Banning on Commercial Surrogacy?
    Don't ban commercial surrogacy, Regulate the industry against exploitation and corrupt practices.

Case 2: SL Story

Wifes age	:	34 years
Husbands age	:	38 years
Marriage	:	8 years
Reason for Surrogacy Treatment	:	3 miscarriages and 2 failed IVF treatment

34 year old wife and 38 year old husband with 8 years of married life presented in June 2014 with history of 3 recurrent miscarriages (all first trimester abortions at 6 weeks.) She had undergone 2 times hystero laparoscopy (telescopic operations) which had revealed left tubal block. Other evaluation pointed out at egg weakness (low AMH) & mild sperm problem. She had 2 unsuccessful IVF (test-tube baby) attempts using donor eggs. This history of 3 recurrent abortions & 2 implantation failures revealed uterine weakness too. So decision of Surrogacy using donor egg &husband's Sperm was taken. Her first Surrogacy cycle gave a possible result. Surrogate mother delivered a healthy baby girl at the end of 9 months.

Case 2: SL Survey

1. Should Commercial Surrogacy Treatment be banned? **Yes/ No**
2. Why did you choose to do Surrogacy? Fashion OR Treatment? **Yes/ No**
3. Every person should have the right to choose the mode for their reproduction? **Agree/ Disagree**
4. Genetic link to the child is important for every human being. **Agree / Disagree**
5. Adoption cannot be forced on couples. **Agree / Disagree**
6. Could a close relative of yours have done Surrogacy for you? **Yes/ No**
7. How should the surrogate mother feel after carrying a baby for you? **Proud/Ashamed**
8. Why you did not adopt a Child?
   Because I am of the opinion that surrogacy is always better than adoption.

9. Please tell us about your life before and after Surrogacy.
   Life was meaningless before surrogacy and post it has changed my life in altogether a different form. Me and my wife has started feeling happiness in true sense.

10. What is your message to the government about **Banning** on Commercial Surrogacy?
    Due respect to law, On my personal opinion, People who can afford, but can't deliver baby due to certain biological challenges can be blessed with gods such a wonderful creation.

Case 3: SM Story

Wifes age	:	**30 years**
Husbands age	:	**32 years**
Marriage	:	**4 years**
Reason for Surrogacy Treatment	:	**Underdeveloped Womb from birth incapable of having periods and carrying a pregnancy**

30 years old wife and 32 years old husband visited the hospital on 2nd December 2015 in view of primary infertility (inability to conceive) since 4 years. She had never had any periods in the past. On performing tests it was detected that she had a very small uterus (womb) from birth.

In 2002, her Laparoscopy (telescopic operation) revealed that her uterus is not capable to carry a pregnancy. So decision of performing surrogacy treatment was taken in February 2016. Fortunately, her ovaries were good and eggs appeared to be strong. Her eggs were grown with injections. After mixing with husband's sperms, resultant embryos (pregnancies) were transferred to surrogate mother. All the procedures were uneventful.

The treatment resulted in twin pregnancy in surrogate mother. Currently the pregnancy is at 7 months without any complications.

Case 3: SM Survey

1. Should commercial surrogacy treatment be banned?   NO

2. Why did you choose to do surrogate ? Fashion OR Treatment ?   NO

3. Every person should have the right to choose the mode for their reproduction ?   Agree

4. Genetic link to the child is important for every human being.   Agree

5. Adoption cannot be forced on couples.   Agree

6. Could a close relative of yours have done Surrogacy for you ?   No

7. How should the surrogate mother feel after carrying a baby for you ?   Proud

8. Why you did not adopt a child ?
   We both want child from our fertility as it was strong for Surrogacy. We also don't want the adopted child to face problem in future as adopted child to be said by people's and also in medical conditions while hospitalized.

9. Please tell us about your life before and after surrogacy .
   Before surrogacy we both have love, peaceful, enjoying and happy life and now after planned for Surrogacy we both are too much have curiosity, love,peaceful, enjoying and happy life and also waiting for the best moment which is going to changed our world. The complete family.

10. What is your message to the government about Banning on Commercial Surrogacy ?
    Government should not ban Surrogacy in our India. It's a good medical technology to those who want there own child from there own fertility. Of course those who can afford. The Surrogacy industry in india doesn't need a ban.

Case 4: VN Story

Wifes age	:	**40 years**
Husbands age	:	**43 years**
Marriage	:	**15 years**
Reason for Surrogacy Treatment	:	**Prolonged treatment, failed IVF attempts and health issues**

40 years old lady and her 43 years old husband visited the hospital on 7th March 2015 with 15 years of childless married life. She had history of one early miscarriage 10 years ago. She had problem of polycystic ovarian disease (hormonal imbalance causing irregular periods). For this reason, she had been aggressively treated with tablets to prepare eggs for almost 18 months and 15 IUI (sperm insemination) cycles. Due to this excessive ovarian stimulation and her age, the quality of her eggs had become poor. This quality was dropping further day by day. This was seen in her blood test, AMH, which was low.

She had undergone one laparoscopy and hysteroscopy(telescopic operation) in 2006, which revealed normal findings. Her previous two attempts of IVF were also failed. Considering this medical background, decision for surrogacy was taken. She decided to use her own eggs despite of low AMH. Couple was very delightful to know positive pregnancy test of surrogate mother and single live pregnancy at 7 weeks of gestation. After uneventful 9 months, surrogate mother delivered a baby girl, thus full filling their dream of parenthood.

Case 4: VN Survey

Here is our opinion:
1. No commercial surrogacy should not be banned.
It is a blessing for couples who cant have their own child.

2. We opted for surrogacy as treatment.

3. We agree that every person must have the choice to choose their method of reproduction.

4. Genetic link with the baby is necessary and important.

5. Adoption cannot be forced on a couple.

6. No. A relative of ours would not have done surrogacy for us.

7. The surrogate mother should feel proud to have carried our baby.
She has given us the joy we so yearned for 16 years. We bless her everyday.

8. We always wanted to have a child of our own. Elders in the family too wanted the genetic link. They have reservations about adoption.

9. We have always been a family couple. We wanted a baby immediately after one year into marriage. But unfortunately it was not happening. We tried all treatments which were not only draining us financial but more importantly emotionally. We had everything but missed having our baby. We started getting depressed to the extent that we found our lives meaningless.
But then surrogacy changed everything. We have been blessed with a baby girl and we are the happiest people on earth. Our lives have changed completely for the good. We look forward to each day with new enthusiasm.
Everyday we bless the surrogate mother and the entire team at Origin for giving us the greatest and the most precious gift.

10. We strongly feel that surrogacy is a blessing. Government should not ban it completely. It will be unfair to couples desiring to have their biological child. Government can set up a criteria if they are bent on making amendments in surrogacy.
Anonymous parents.

Case 5: RP Story

Wifes age	:	**31 years**
Husbands age	:	**32 years**
Marriage	:	**8 years**
Reason for Surrogacy Treatment	:	**Severe health condition on strong medications**

31 year old female & 32 year old male consulted the medical experts in June 2014 with 8 years of married life & inability to conceive. Husband had mild sperm problem & wife had low AMH (egg weakness.) Also she was known case of ulcerative colitis for which she was on steroids & Immunosuppressive therapy. She had underwent IVF treatment in 2012 which resulted in twin pregnancy, but unfortunately she had preterm delivery at 6 months and the babies could not survive. Considering her health issue & uterine problem, decision of surrogacy with her own eggs and husband's sperm was taken. This gave a positive result in the first attempt. Couple was happy to be parents of a healthy baby boy, at the end of 9 months.

Dr. Sandeep Mane

Case 5: RP Survey

1. Should Commercial Surrogacy Treatment be banned? ~~Yes~~/ No
2. Why did you choose to do Surrogacy? Fashion OR Treatment?

   Treatment

3. Every person should have the right to choose the mode for their reproduction?

   Agree/ ~~Disagree~~

4. Genetic link to the child is important for every human being. Agree / ~~Disagree~~

5. Adoption cannot be forced on couples. Agree / ~~Disagree~~
6. Could a close relative of yours have done Surrogacy for you? ~~Yes~~/ No
7. How should the surrogate mother feel after carrying a baby for you?

   Proud/~~Ashamed~~

8. Why you did not adopt a Child?
   Adoption of a child was a last option for us. When there is an option available to us where we can have a biological child why not go for it. Mentally we are happier when the child borne is ours rather through adoption.

9. Please tell us about your life before and after Surrogacy.

   We had being trying for a baby for almost 8 years. We went through all possible procedures from simplest to the most complicated process like IUI, ICSI, IVF. We did not achieve the desired result through the above mentioned methods. We were left with only 2 options viz. adoption or surrogacy.

   Initially surrogacy was very difficult to digest as we believed how the society would react to our decision. In fact we were the first in our entire family to have a baby in this format. But then we decided to go for surrogacy. Once we took the decision, life was far simpler for us. Now we were completely relaxed and happily waiting for the arrival of the baby.

   Then came the date we were eagerly waiting for.. 14.5.2015. We were blessed with a baby boy. We cannot express the joy and happiness we feeling that day. Life got completed for us on 14.05.2015. There cannot be any special day for us other than the day we took ZIAAN in our hands. Today we are in a state of mind that we were never before ZIAAN came in our life. Life has changed completely for us and we would like to thank Dr. Mane for this. Life has more meaning for us now.

10. What is your message to the government about Banning on Commercial Surrogacy?

    Commercial surrogacy should not be banned at all. Practically no close family member turns up for being a surrogate mother. If the government is intending to put a ban on commercial surrogacy for the reason that surrogate mothers are being exploited, the government can have guidelines or rules to be followed for it. But, surely there cannot any reason to ban surrogacy for a childless couple.

Case 6: MP Story

Wifes age	:	35 years
Husbands age	:	35 years
Marriage	:	4 years
Reason for Surrogacy Treatment	:	**Prolonged treatment with repeated failures**

35 years old lady and 35 years old husband with 4 years of married life consulted the hospital in October 2014.

She had low AMH value indicating weak eggs. She had undergone 2 cycles of advanced IVF treatment in the past, which had failed.

The couple was advised OD surrogacy treatment. In second attempt, surrogate mother tested positive for pregnancy. Ultrasound on her revealed twin pregnancy which was reduced to singleton at 12 weeks. Surrogate mother delivered a baby girl after 9 months uneventfully.

Case 6: MP Survey

1. Should Commercial Surrogacy Treatment be banned? **No**
2. Why did you choose to do Surrogacy? **Treatment**
3. Every person should have the right to choose the mode for their reproduction? **Agree**
4. Genetic link to the child is important for every human being. **Agree**
5. Adoption cannot be forced on couples. **Agree**
6. Could a close relative of yours have done Surrogacy for you? **Yes**
7. How should the surrogate mother feel after carrying a baby for you? **Proud**
8. Why you did not adopt a Child?
   _Adoption is the last resort. As far as possible we wanted our own genetic tradition to continue in our child.
9. Please tell us about your life before and after Surrogacy.
   _We had almost lost hope that we will be blessed with our own child. After surrogacy our life is full of happimess and gratitude towards God, our doctor and ofcourse the new advances of science. _____
10. What is your message to the government about **Banning** on Commercial Surrogacy?
    _There is no need to completely ban surrogacy as long as it is voluntary and ethical in every sense of the word. However it should be a transparent and carefully carried out process.

Case 7: SR Story

Wifes age	:	33 years
Husbands age	:	40 years
Marriage	:	6 years
Reason for Surrogacy Treatment	:	Severe health condition on strong medications

In May 2016, 33 year old wife & 40 year old husband approached the hospital for their desire to have a second child. They were married since 6 years & had 3 year old daughter. After delivery of her daughter 3 years ago by cesarean section, she developed breathing difficulty & swelling over body – 6 weeks post-delivery. She was diagnosed to have dilated cardiomyopathy (reduced cardiac function) with ejection fraction of 20%. She recovered slowly with medical management. Though she recovered from this peripartum cardiomyopathy, cardiac physician has explained very high chance of recurrence of similar episode in subsequent pregnancy. Thus carrying pregnancy herself was very risky. So they decided to go for gestational surrogacy with her eggs & husband's sperm. After IVF treatment, surrogate mother tested positive for pregnancy. Sonography revealed singleton healthy baby. Currently she is in the 6th month carrying pregnancy uneventfully.

Case 7: SR Survey

1. Should Commercial Surrogacy Treatment be banned? Yes/ No
   No

2. Why did you choose to do Surrogacy? Fashion OR Treatment? Yes/ No
   Treatment

3. Every person should have the right to choose the mode for their reproduction?
   Agree/ Disagree

   Agree

4. Genetic link to the child is important for every human being. Agree / Disagree

   Agree

5. Adoption cannot be forced on couples. Agree / Disagree
   Agree

6. Could a close relative of yours have done Surrogacy for you? Yes/ No
   No

7. How should the surrogate mother feel after carrying a baby for you?

   Proud/Ashamed

   Proud

8. Why you did not adopt a Child?
   We already have one child of our own. We want to have one more child of our own, so we never chose adoption as an option.

9. Please tell us about your life before and after Surrogacy.
   My wife developed a rare heart condition called PeriPartum Cardiomyopathy after delivery of our first baby. Her heart became so weak that it reached a life threatening stage. She finally survived due to her strong will power. All the expert gynecologists and cardiologists advised us not to have another child because there are high chances of this condition reoccurring and it could prove fatal. Our life was shattered with the thought of not been able to have another child. My wife almost went into depression and we very feeling that pain every single moment. Gestational Surrogacy came as a ray of hope that we can have our own baby without risking the life of my wife.

Case 8: SS Story

Wifes age	:	38 years
Husbands age	:	38 years
Marriage	:	8 years
Reason for Surrogacy Treatment	:	**Severe health condition and uterine problems**

38 years old wife and her 38 year old husband were taking fertility treatment at the hospital since 2008. Over a period of 8 years, she had 4 miscarriages. She had a problem of polycystic ovarian disease with egg weakness (low AMH) and right tubal block. She was also suffering from hypertension(raised blood pressure). Her BP was controlled on antihypertensive medication. Husband had problem of coarctation of aorta. He had undergone angioplasty followed by cardiac surgery in 2008. She had undergone 12 IUI cycles which had failed. Also she had 4 unsuccessful IVF attempts, first with own eggs followed by donor eggs. To improve uterine functionality, new technologies like instilling GCSF solution was used but unfortunately pregnancy could not go beyond 6 weeks. Considering uterine factor & egg weakness, treatment plan with donor egg surrogacy was suggested. Currently surrogate mother is 12 weeks pregnant and will carry a singleton pregnancy.

Case 8: SS Survey

1. Should Commercial Surrogacy Treatment be banned? Yes/ ~~No~~
2. Why did you choose to do Surrogacy? ~~Fashion~~ OR Treatment? Yes/ No
3. Every person should have the right to choose the mode for their reproduction? Agree/ ~~Disagree~~
4. Genetic link to the child is important for every human being. ~~Agree~~/ Disagree
5. Adoption cannot be forced on couples. Agree/ ~~Disagree~~
6. Could a close relative of yours have done Surrogacy for you? ~~Yes~~/ No
7. How should the surrogate mother feel after carrying a baby for you? Proud/ ~~Ashamed~~
8. Why you did not adopt a Child?
   The procedure is too stringent. We have applied in Apr'16 but the waiting period is too long. And looking at the stringent laws being introduced every time for adoption, the waiting period is never going to end.

9. Please tell us about your life before and after Surrogacy.
   We have been married for around 11 years by now. Continual fertility treatment for years have brought mental, physical and financial trauma to the entire family. Surrogacy has come as a boon to us even though the expenses are high. But at least we have a hope here that we will not be childless anymore.

10. What is your message to the government about **Banning** on Commercial Surrogacy?
    Ban on commercial surrogacy should be well thought of. Government should go through the case studies before taking a decision. Banning commercial surrogacy is definitely not a solution to the exploitation of surrogate mothers by some hospitals. Hospitals should be graded and committees should be assigned to keep an eye on such incidents so that banning of surrogacy can be done at hospital/physician level and not at the national level.

Case 9: NS Story

Wifes age	:	30 years
Husbands age	:	40 years
Marriage	:	9 years
Reason for Surrogacy Treatment	:	Severe health condition on strong medications with prolonged failure of advanced IVF treatment

30 year old female & 40 year old male with 9 years of married life & prolonged suffering of infertility visited the hospital in February 2014. Wife was suffering from connective tissue disorder – SLF (Systemic lupus erythematosus.) She was on steroids & immunosuppressive therapy and still used to have active spells of disease like severe Arthritis. She had history of genital tuberculosis which had damaged her left tube (left hydrosalpinx.) Her hysterolaparoscopy had revealed too many bowel adhesions. She had undergone 4 unsuccessful IVF attempts. In 2012, she conceived, but unfortunately the pregnancy was in the damaged left tube (ectopic pregnancy). This is a dangerous condition and hence the tube had to be removed along with the pregnancy. This was an open operation due to the risk to her life. The decision to perform surrogacy had to be taken because of her high risk background, weak eggs, abnormal tube & repeated IVF failures. Currently the treatment process is ongoing.

Case 9 : NS Survey

1. Should Commercial Surrogacy Treatment be banned? ⟶ <u>No</u>

2. Why did you choose to do Surrogacy? Fashion OR Treatment? ⟶ <u>Yes Treatment</u>

3. Every person should have the right to choose the mode for their reproduction? ⟶ Agree

4. Genetic link to the child is important for every human being. ⟶ Agree

5. Adoption cannot be forced on couples. ⟶ Agree

6. Could a close relative of yours have done Surrogacy for you? ⟶ No

7. How should the surrogate mother feel after carrying a baby for you?

    ⟶ Proud

8. Why you did not adopt a Child?

    Because we want Our Own Child.

9. Please tell us about your life before and after Surrogacy.

    Our Life is going well till now. And after child it will become more happy, joyous & auspicious.

10. What is your message to the government about Banning on Commercial Surrogacy?

    This treatment gives us one hope to fulfill our wish. Therefore I request you that please do not stop Commercial Surrogacy treatment.

Please do not disclose my identity.

Case 10: SU Story

Wifes age	:	35 years
Husbands age	:	37 years
Marriage	:	8 years
Reason for Surrogacy Treatment	:	**Severe health condition with recurrent (4 times) pregnancy loss**

35 years old lady and her 37 years old husband approached the hospital in May 2013. This couple had numerous pregnancies, but then had miscarriages repeatedly. There were 4 miscarriages at 14 weeks of gestation indicating incompetent OS (weakness of the neck of the womb). She had fibroid uterus and right unhealthy fallopian tube (hydrosalphinx) for which she had undergone hysterolaparoscopy (telescopic operation to remove the lump), with myomectomy. Post procedure, IVF attempt resulted in twin pregnancy but miscarriage happened again at 14 weeks. Meanwhile she was diagnosed to have hypercoagulability of blood (increased clotting in the blood, which can be a life threatening condition. Due to this medical background and weak eggs (low AMH), she underwent two gestational surrogacy attempts which were unsuccessful.

The couple was offered OD Surrogacy treatment which was successful in her 4th attempt.

Case 10: SU Survey

1. Should Commercial Surrogacy Treatment be banned? **NO**

2. Why did you choose to do Surrogacy? Fashion OR Treatment? **Treatment**

3. Every person should have the right to choose the mode for their reproduction? **Agree**

4. Genetic link to the child is important for every human being. **Disagree**

5. Adoption cannot be forced on couples. **Agree**6. Could a close relative of yours have done Surrogacy for you? **No**

6. Could a close relative of yours have done Surrogacy for you? **NO**

7. How should the surrogate mother feel after carrying a baby for you? **Proud**

8. Why you did not adopt a Child?
We were planning to adopt child and had already started the Process

9. Please tell us about your life before and after Surrogacy.
Due to medical complications we were not able to conceive and carry our child therefore we opted for surrogacy and we are lucky to be blessed with a beautiful son who has filled our life with happiness and motivation. Life before our son was exploring our options and avenue to have kid and wishing for one. Now after having him, we are happy and wish that people are blessed with options to explore to have kids if they want

10. .What is your message to the government about **Banning** on Commercial Surrogacy?
Please do not make decisions about others life. Government can guide and address their concerns differently rather then ban and taking away peoples option to have family.

Case 11: SV Story

Wifes age	:	43 years
Husbands age	:	45 years
Marriage	:	12 years
Reason for Surrogacy Treatment	:	**Recurrent failure of advanced treatment with uterine problems**

A Couple of 12 year history of childlessness approached the hospital in March 2016 for fertility treatment. Wife is 43 years old and husband is 45 years age with 13 years of married life. She had history of genital tuberculosis in the past. Over period of these 12 years, she had undergone laparoscopy (telescopic operation) thrice and hysteroscopy twice. Hysteroscopy had revealed adhesions (bands) inside uterine cavity (Asherman's syndrome). Adhesiolysis procedure was done to break the bands and improve the womb. She had undergone IUI cycles 12 times which had failed. She had 3 unsuccessful attempts of IVF cycles with own eggs and one unsuccessful attempt of gestational surrogacy till now. She had developed weak eggs (egg factor). Still she wanted to give one more chance to self-eggs. The first attempt of gestational surrogacy has failed. So decision of OD surrogacy was taken. After the treatment cycle, Surrogate mother tested positive for pregnancy currently pregnancy is ongoing.

Case 11: SV Survey

1. Should Commercial Surrogacy Treatment be banned?　　　Yes/ **No** ✓
2. Why did you choose to do Surrogacy? Fashion OR **Treatment** ✓?　　Yes/ No
3. Every person should have the right to choose the mode for their reproduction?　　　**Agree** ✓/ Disagree
4. Genetic link to the child is important for every human being. **Agree** ✓ / Disagree
5. Adoption cannot be forced on couples.　　　**Agree** ✓ / Disagree
6. Could a close relative of yours have done Surrogacy for you?　　Yes/ **No** ✓
7. How should the surrogate mother feel after carrying a baby for you? **Proud** ✓ /Ashamed
8. Why you did not adopt a Child?
   In order to give genetic link to child

9. Please tell us about your life before and after Surrogacy.
   After undergoing various fertility treatment (IVF, IUI) Surrogacy was only solution. Surrogacy has given us new hopes in our life to fulfill our dreams to have our own child.

10. What is your message to the government about **Banning** on Commercial Surrogacy?
    → We feel surrogacy is a boon to couples who are unable to bear child due to various infertility problems
    → By banning Commercial Surrogacy, Govt is killing hopes of many childless couples.
    → Just because few celebrities are opting Commercial Surrogacy as fashion & statement, banning it is an injustice to lakhs of childless couples.

Case 12: Mrs Sonali Hemraj Jaiswal Story

Wifes age	: 39 years
Huisbands age	: 44 years
Marriage	: 17 years
Reason for Surrogacy Treatment	: Multiple IVF failures and advancing age

This pleasant couple visited the hospital in 2010 with history of 5 failed prior attempts at IVF treatment. They had also undergone numerous IUI treatment cycles and were exhausted. At our hospital, they tried two more attempts, including surrogacy, but were unsuccessful. Finally, in September 2014, the Surrogacy treatment cycle was successful. This resulted in a baby girl at full term. They are very grateful to the surrogate mother who has helped them to fulfill their dreams.

Case 12: Mrs Sonali Hemraj Jaiswal Story

This couple marries for over 10 years underwent numerous IVF treatments and finally got this baby girl via surrogacy treatment.

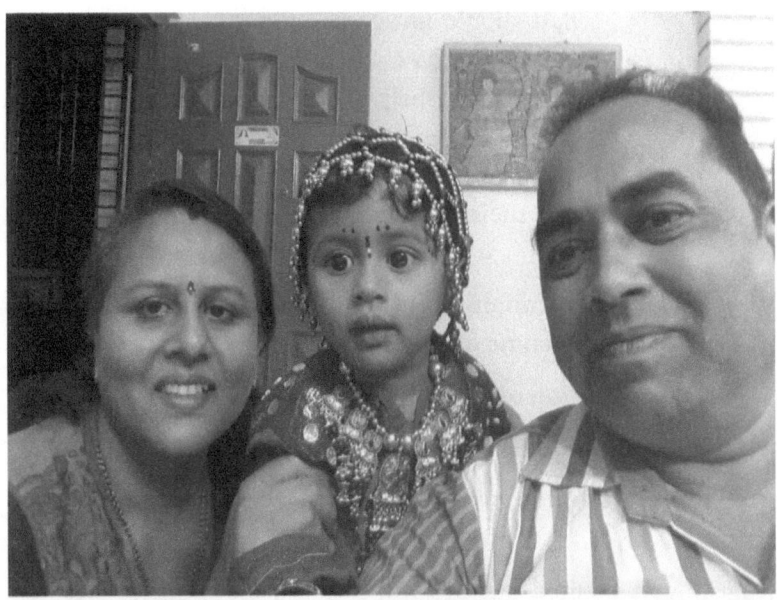

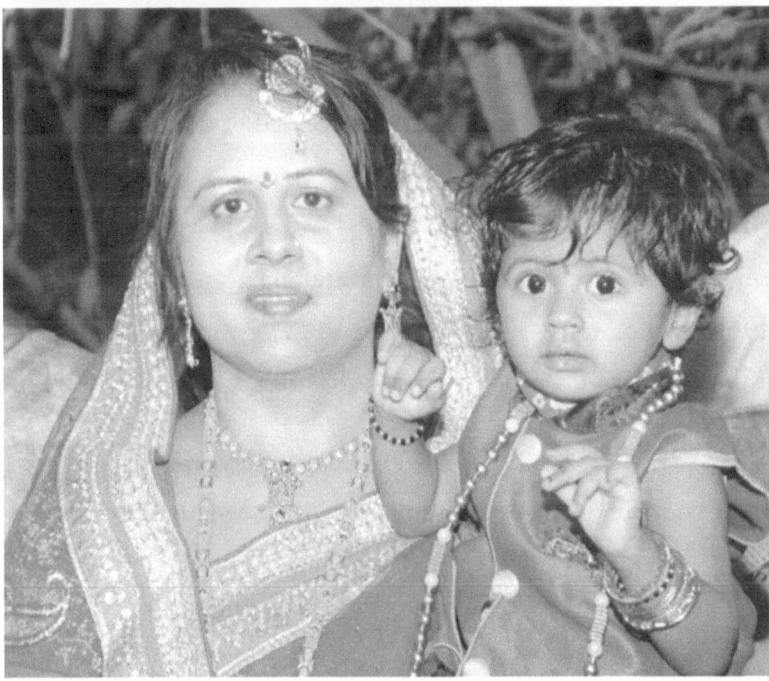

SURROGATE MOTHERS- Their Stories and Opinions

Name: Mrs. Faimida Shaikh **Age: 26yrs**

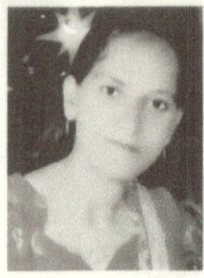

According to me in accordance to the new surrogacy bill, it should not be banned. This will adversely going to affect our lives. My family is going through financial crisis, with the help of surrogacy. I am helping my family as well as trying to give a bright future to my children. Instead of doing some bad deeds, we help someone to fulfill their dreams. What else will bless me than this help!!!

Opinion: Please, Government has to think on whether to ban surrogacy or not. This is a best income option for us.

Please give your opinion on upcoming Surrogacy Bill?

Request the Government not to ban surrogacy option.

If Surrogacy gets banned, what type of work you will do to fulfill your basic needs?

If surrogacy gets banned our life will become more difficult as that will enforce me to do some labor work or housekeeper's job.

What problems made you to take a decision for Surrogacy?

For my child's education purpose I have decided to do surrogacy.

Do you feel ashamed of doing Surrogacy?

No. I don't feel so.

Do you feel that you are being get exploited by doing a Surrogacy?

No, absolutely not in this Hospital. I don't have any idea about other centre.

What message you would wish to give our Government regarding Surrogacy Bill?

Government has to rethink about this surrogacy bill. They have to think about our poor conditions, educational status and our helplessness.

Name: Bisna Rokay Age: 34yrs

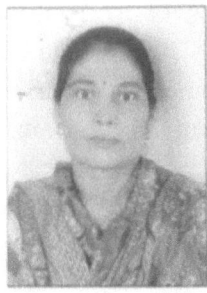

Surrogacy has to be continued. It gives great help to poor people. If surrogacy gets banned, we will have to do farming on uncultivated lands, ultimately we are not going to get money. To repay our loans I have decided to do surrogacy. In rural areas, people are not aware of about surrogacy. But for me it is a good work as per my experience.

Opinion: Surrogacy should be continued. It is not a shameful work.

Please give your opinion on upcoming Surrogacy Bill?

Surrogacy has to be continued. As it helps us.

If Surrogacy gets banned, what type of work you will do to fulfill your basic needs?

No other work than farming. The income from farming is not that enough to fulfill our needs.

What problems made you to take a decision for Surrogacy?

We have debts to repay hence to give a financial support to my husband, I have taken this decision.

Do you feel ashamed of doing Surrogacy?

No. But in rural areas they think it in a wrong way.

Do you feel that you are being get exploited by doing a Surrogacy?

No, absolutely not, instead it gives money and good wishes.

What message you would wish to give our Government regarding Surrogacy Bill?

This is a good deed we do for someone, who is not able to give a birth to a child due to some medical and physical inabilities. We are just the source for their joy.

Name: Pabitra Thapa   **Age: 30yrs**

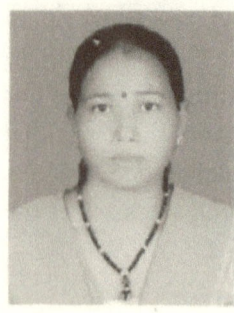

I have poor economic conditions. We have taken debts from landlords for building our small own house. The amount is huge and hence I wanted to help my husband to give a financial support. By doing Surrogacy I am getting big lump sum amount, so have decided to it. It is wrong to say that someone gets exploited by doing Surrogacy, as my experience was so good. Government has to make people aware of Surrogacy they have to think about us before doing ban.

Opinion: Please give your opinion on upcoming Surrogacy Bill?

Surrogacy should not be banned.

If Surrogacy gets banned, what type of work you will do to fulfill your basic needs?

If surrogacy get banned then no any other good option for me for earning money.

What problems made you to take a decision for Surrogacy?

I have dream of my own house due to this I am doing surrogacy.

Do you feel ashamed of doing Surrogacy?

No. but lack of awareness outside related to surrogacy so sometime feels shameful, because they are taking it wrongly.

Do you feel that you are being get exploited by doing a Surrogacy?

No, I don't feel so.

What message you would wish to give our Government regarding Surrogacy Bill?

Surrogacy should not be banned. Government have to rethink on it.

Name: Mrs. Khushi Sunar [use photo] **Age: 24yrs**

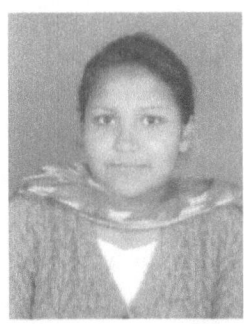

Surrogacy should not be banned. I am from poor class family. I am an illiterate person. I have responsibility of my son and my parents, for their better future I have choose this way for earning money. I am quite satisfied after taking such decision. I am feeling homely environment in this hospital. So I do not think that this is a shameful work or we don't get exploited through this work.

Opinion: Whether Government going to ban such a good deed., then what is the alternate way for us.

Please give your opinion on upcoming Surrogacy Bill?

Surrogacy should not be banned by Government.

If Surrogacy gets banned, what type of work you will do to fulfill your basic needs?

I am an illiterate person so any other work will not fulfill our basic needs.

What problems made you to take a decision for Surrogacy?

I am alone with my child, so I have decided to do surrogacy for our better future.

Do you feel ashamed of doing Surrogacy?

No.

Do you feel that you are being get exploited by doing a Surrogacy?

No, I don't feel so.

What message you would wish to give our Government regarding Surrogacy Bill?

Whether Government going to ban such a good deed., then what is the alternate way for us.

Name: Mrs. K S　　　　　　　　　　　　　　　**Age: 24yrs**

According to me Surrogacy should not be banned. If Surrogacy will get banned, I would rather have to do a labor work as I am an illiterate person. My financial condition is very poor. I have no any other support. For bright future of my children's as a responsible parent, I am striving hard to give them good facilities and hence Surrogacy is good option for me. Surrogacy is not exploitation, rather I feel it is a great work we do.

Opinion: If Government is going to ban Surrogacy, please give us other better options of income to get money in bulk.

Please give your opinion on upcoming Surrogacy Bill?

Surrogacy should not be banned.

If Surrogacy gets banned, what type of work you will do to fulfill your basic needs?

As I am an uneducated person, I would have preferred to do labor work.

What problems made you to take a decision for Surrogacy?

We do not have any source of income hence for my children better future I have chosen to do surrogacy.

Do you feel ashamed of doing Surrogacy?

No, I do not feel ashamed of doing this.

Do you feel that you are being get exploited by doing a Surrogacy?

No, Surrogacy is not an exploitation for me.

What message you would wish to give our Government regarding Surrogacy Bill?

We are poor needy people. If surrogacy gets banned we will not get lump sum amount by any other source of income.

Name: Mrs. KB   **Age: 24yrs**

As per my opinion, surrogacy is a noble work. It should not be banned instead it has to be regulated with well defined rules. Surrogacy is a good option of income. I am less educated and belong to low poverty background. Me & my family wishes to have our own house. It is our dream. Hence I have decided to do a surrogacy to contribute towards building my dream. It is not a shameful work, but mostly in rural areas people have many misunderstandings about this.

Opinion: We majority of lower income group women earn by way of surrogacy, hence Surrogacy should not be banned.

Please give your opinion on upcoming Surrogacy Bill?

Such a good work - Surrogacy should not be banned by Government.

If Surrogacy gets banned, what type of work you will do to fulfill your basic needs?

There is no other option than working as a maid.

What problems made you to take a decision for Surrogacy?

For having own house I have taken this decision. And also to support my family as husband's salary is very less.

Do you feel ashamed of doing Surrogacy?

No, I do not feel ashamed of doing this, but people are not aware of this.

Do you feel that you are being get exploited by doing a Surrogacy?

No, I don't feel so.

What message you would wish to give our Government regarding Surrogacy Bill?

No, it should not be banned. Now a day many women choose this option.

Name: Mrs. RP   **Age: 28yrs**

Surrogacy is not a shameful work but it's a good deed we do for someone. According to me, as per my experience surrogacy is not exploitation. Though Government is saying it is exploitation, it is not the only sector where exploitation occurs. It exists at every level in the society. Is prostitution is not exploitation? Working at someone's home as housekeeper or as a maid and doing so many bad things under their pressure, isn't it exploitation? With proper rules & regulation surrogacy has to be continued for people like us as an income option to fulfill our responsibilities.

Opinion: If government is planning to ban surrogacy, whether the Government is will assure that they will give us another better option of income or else they are closing our income source.

Please give your opinion on upcoming Surrogacy Bill?

Surrogacy should not be banned by Government. It is a good deed.

If Surrogacy gets banned, what type of work you will do to fulfill your basic needs?

I am an illiterate person so any other work will not fulfill our basic needs.

What problems made you to take a decision for Surrogacy?

My husband is jobless and we have debts to repay, so I have decided to do surrogacy.

Do you feel ashamed of doing Surrogacy?

No.

Do you feel that you are being get exploited by doing a Surrogacy?

No, I don't feel so.

What message you would wish to give our Government regarding Surrogacy Bill?

No, it should not be banned. Is the Government is going to take our responsibilities or provide us any other employment option.

Name: MS   **Age: 28yrs**

A Surrogate mother of 28 years old says, Surrogacy is a good option for us to earn income. If Surrogacy will get banned, as we are poor and uneducated people I will have to work at someone's house as a maid or as a housekeeper. To give better education to my children I have decided to do a Surrogacy. No, I have not been exploited by any means in the hospital where I did Surrogacy. Every one there was so good, caring and helping. Government has to give better option of earnings to us before applying ban on Surrogacy.

Opinion: Please give your opinion on upcoming Surrogacy Bill?

Surrogacy should not be banned, but it's continued with proper rules and regulations.

If Surrogacy gets banned, what type of work you will do to fulfill your basic needs?

According to me surrogacy is a good work but if surrogacy get ban then I have to do labor work or housekeeper work.

What problems made you to take a decision for Surrogacy?

For my child's education I have taken this surrogacy decision.

Do you feel ashamed of doing Surrogacy?

No. instead I tell to everybody about my surrogacy.

Do you feel that you are being get exploited by doing a Surrogacy?

No, absolutely not, my experience of this hospital throughout 9 months is very good.

What message you would wish to give our Government regarding Surrogacy Bill?

Surrogacy should not be banned otherwise Government should give answer that what should we do?

Name: NP **Age: 28yrs**

I am a helpless woman who is searching an opportunity which can help me for resolve my money problem. Before starting of this surrogacy procedure I have done work in bureau but I can't earn as much as my requirement. So that I have taken surrogacy decision and now I am satisfied. According to me, as per my experience surrogacy is not exploitation or a shameful work. It is a good deed, due to which we can help someone who is in deep need. What else will bless me than this help!!!

Opinion: Surrogacy should not be banned. Government has to think about infertile couple because this option is helpful for completing their dream.

Please give your opinion on upcoming Surrogacy Bill?

Surrogacy should be continued.

If Surrogacy gets banned, what type of work you will do to fulfill your basic needs?

If surrogacy get be banned then no any other good option for me I have to do labor work only.

What problems made you to take a decision for Surrogacy?

I am staying alone with my child. I have dream of my own house due to this I am doing surrogacy.

Do you feel ashamed of doing Surrogacy?

No. but lack of awareness outside related to surrogacy.

Do you feel that you are being get exploited by doing a Surrogacy?

No, I don't feel so.

What message you would wish to give our Government regarding Surrogacy Bill?

Surrogacy should not be banned. Government has to think about infertile couple. Because this option is helpful for them.

Name: Mrs. KW   **Age: 23yrs**

Surrogacy should not be banned. If Surrogacy will get banned, I would rather have to do a labor work as I am an illiterate person. My financial condition is very poor. I have to repay our debts. It is not a shameful work, but mostly in rural areas people have many misunderstandings about this. So government has to give information in rural area about surrogacy and help us and a couple who are in need.

Opinion: If government is planning to ban surrogacy, whether the Government is will assure that they will give us another better option of income or else they are closing our income source.

Please give your opinion on upcoming Surrogacy Bill?

Surrogacy should not be banned by Government.

If Surrogacy gets banned, what type of work you will do to fulfill your basic needs?

I am an illiterate person so any other work will not fulfill our basic needs.

What problems made you to take a decision for Surrogacy?

We have debts to repay, so I have decided to do surrogacy.

Do you feel ashamed of doing Surrogacy?

No.

Do you feel that you are being get exploited by doing a Surrogacy?

No, I don't feel so.

What message you would wish to give our Government regarding Surrogacy Bill?

All poor class people like us has requirements are lot and due to this surrogacy should be continue. It is not a crime. So why Government is trying to ban it we are unable to know. Our family future seems to be dark now.

Chapter 4

Surrogacy – Currently Compensatory Altruistic Not Commercial

Over the years, surrogacy has been a life changing treatment for thousands of couples who suffered enormously in their lives due to prolonged fertility treatment. It has been a boon to so many couples who are now enjoying the pleasures of a family. The treatment has also helped the young women who were in need of money for their personal reasons. The growing number of women coming forward to do surrogacy and the number of intended parents taking this treatment is a proof in itself that the process has been liked by both parties. This treatment was completed successfully in all these years even without any legislation in place. Credit must be given to the surrogate mothers and the intended parents for their sincerity in the treatment. It was the lack of available legislation, which led to some complications and allowed some clinicians to offer the treatment as per their own choices.

The international community pounced on the irregularities and tarnished the image of this treatment. Other countries of the world had their own reasons for banning surrogacy, but they could not accept the successful model in India. They became mere spectators of the massive success. It became very embarrassing for them to see their citizens flocking to India and returning home as happy families. India had carved a place for itself. This was a result of our population changes, availability of internationally trained good doctors, the latest technology and the medical facilities at par or even better than anywhere in the world. It was this very success that led to the global community to criticize this treatment and they started calling it names- rent a womb, baby farms, baby factory and so on…

Many states of America and Russia continue to offer surrogacy even today at three times the cost in India. They never heeded to such criticism. India took too much notice of these voices against surrogacy and rushed into taking action against this treatment. This happened because there are very few people to speak in favour of this treatment. Many fear that they may get targeted by the opponents of surrogacy. The intended parents do not wish to come out in the open and express their positive feelings and the surrogate mothers are generally not very capable of voicing their opinions. The sporadic cases involving celebrities triggered media coverage on the subject. The positive stories did not get so much attention and hence a biased view got created, "The rich exploiting the poor in an unregulated business of human lives." Even today, very few people understand what surrogacy means, what is actually done, how it is done and the issues involved

Problems were there. Regulation was definitely needed, because the treatment had reached mammoth proportions and too much freedom was not good. Each time a bad incident occurred, the media covered the story. Each bad incident taught a new lesson and further regulations were designed. Good changes were being made to stop all problems. Initially, there were no regulations and any patient would come to India from any country and request treatment. The Indian government took control of this situation step by step. In 2012, there was a ban imposed on surrogacy for the same sex couples and single parents from abroad. In 2014, all foreigners were banned and in 2016, a complete ban on commercial surrogacy in India has been proposed.

Surrogacy came into the limelight for reasons as outlined below. There must be many more high profile cases of surrogacy, but the following ones were noted with prominence in the recent years.

The International Stories that Hit the Headlines Criticizing Surrogacy

2008: Case 1–Baby Manjhi Yamada. This Japanese couple filed for divorce during their surrogacy treatment before the baby was born. Japanese law did not recognize surrogacy and Indian law did not allow a single man to adopt a baby. Baby was later handed over to her grandmother Emiko. She took care of the child and got a travel certificate after two months.

Solution to avoid this: Only offer surrogacy treatment to couples whose country allows surrogacy and take written confirmation from the country that the baby will be allowed to go back to its home country. Couples should make enforceable agreement in which they give clear instructions about what happens in case of divorce and allocate responsibility to a named guardian.

2010: Case 2–Israeli father of twins born to Indian surrogate mother denied permission to bring sons home. DNA test for paternity was asked by the Israeli courts, which was then done.

Solution: The issue of same sex couples needs to be addressed by the honorable courts and such treatment must ONLY be undertaken if there is clear permission in the law of the country to which the intended parents belong. Until such clarity is obtained, surrogacy should not be undertaken for those international patients, because issues may arise later.

2010: Case 3–A German couple had twin babies via surrogacy in India. The babies were eventually allowed to return to Germany, where they were adopted by their parents as per the German rules.

Solution: Only offer surrogacy treatment to couples whose country allows surrogacy and take written confirmation from the country that the baby will be allowed to go back to its home country.

2012: Case 4–Australian couple abandoned surrogate born son with downs syndrome in India and only took the twin sister.

Solution: Legally enforceable agreement should cover all these possible scenarios. It must be binding on the couple to abide by the agreement.

The three celebrity cases that brought surrogacy into the limelight were:

2011: Case 5 A bollywood filmstar declared that he had a baby born via surrogacy for reasons as advised by his doctor. He has children from before and had another child for his personal reasons. This is currently being criticized, because couples with previous children, even from previous marriages are being banned from having children via surrogacy according to the new bill.

Solution: The honorable courts should decide if this ban infringes on the persons human rights and whether the constitution gives him the right to do so. Legal opinion should clarify this situation. Such treatment can only be done in future if it has been given legal permission.

2013: Case 6 Another bollywood filmstar declared that he had a baby born via surrogacy. He also had previous children and chose to have a third child for his personal reasons.

Solution: The honorable courts should decide if this ban infringes on the persons human rights and whether the constitution gives him the right to do so. Legal opinion should clarify this situation. Such treatment can only be done in future if it has been given legal permission.

2016: Case 7 One more bollywood filmstar had a child through surrogacy. He chose to do it as a single father and prompted different reactions from people.

Solution: The honorable courts should give clear guidelines about who can and who cannot undertake surrogacy. Legal opinion should clarify this situation. Such treatment can only be done in future if it has been given legal permission.

It would be good to face the issues head-on rather than dodging them or squashing them. International couples are faced with different issues and these can be easily addressed by proper law that helps the clinicians to offer this treatment to international couples without repeating the mistakes of the past. If this just seems impossible to manage, ban is obviously the last step that may become necessary. The issue of single parents, surrogacy for fashion, surrogacy by people with previous children are all easily dealt with by defining the eligibility criteria. This will be a legal decision on the basis of human and constitutional rights. These were all avoidable. Regulation would have avoided almost all the above problems that happened during surrogacy.

Chapter 5

Regulation for Surrogacy – 2005 to 2014

The incidence of infertility has increased significantly all over the world. 10 to 15% couples worldwide are infertile. In India alone, almost 20 million couples suffered from infertility. This led to mushrooming of fertility clinics and hospitals across the country. Legal complications were bound to happen as there was lack of regulation to control the treatment.

The Indian Council for Medical Research (ICMR) was given the responsibility of framing the guidelines with consultation of various stake holders. In the UK, in such situations where the government is concerned about a particular medical matter, it consults the appropriate Royal College and arrives at decisions. In the case of surrogacy in India, there is no single responsible body with whom the consultation could happen about regulating this treatment.

The process of formulating a bill and eventually a law is a long drawn path and it started with the formation of a committee aimed at bringing the required regulations. The guidelines were prepared in 2005 and reviewed from time to time over the subsequent years, **(Chart 10)**. In 2014, it had almost been finalized for cabinet submission. The guidelines were expected to be followed, but did not have full legal standing.

Chart 10: Surrogacy for Whom ??... ART bill overview from 2005 to 2016

	Single parent, same sex couples – Foreigners	Foreigners	Indian citizens	OCI, PIO, NRI, Foreigner married to Indian citizen	Single parent, same sex couples - Indian
2005	Allowed with regulations	Allowed with regulations	Allowed with regulations	Allowed with regulations	Allowed with regulations
2012	Ban	Allowed with regulations	Allowed with regulations	Allowed with regulations	Allowed with regulations
2014		Ban	Allowed with regulations	Allowed with regulations	Allowed with regulations
2016			Ban	Ban	Ban

Chart 11: Changes in Surrogacy Bill in India

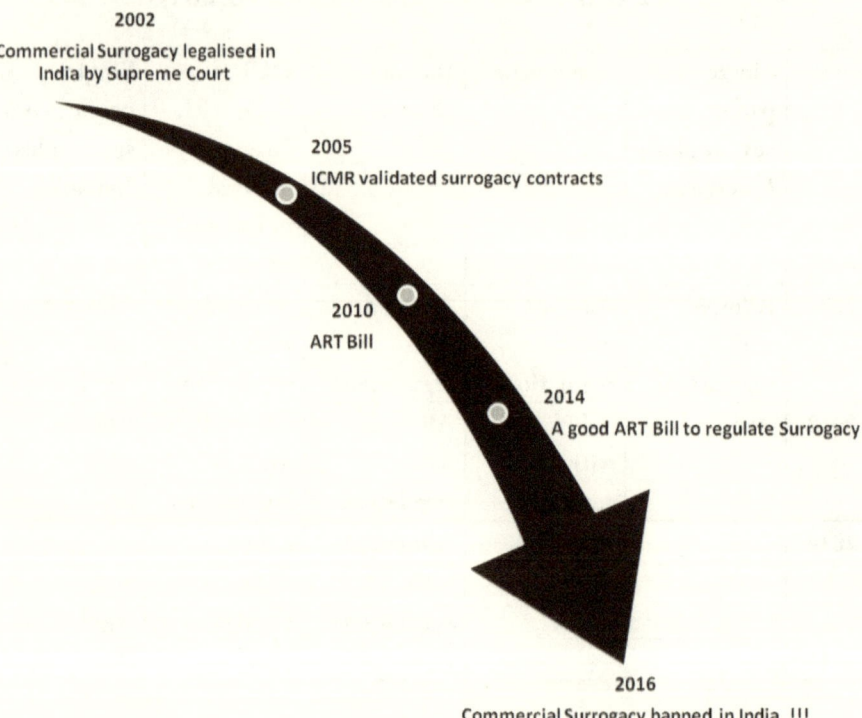

The Journey from Regulation to Ban on Surrogacy was as Follows (Chart 11)

2005: National Guidelines for Accreditation, Supervision and Regulation of ART Clinics in India

- By extensive consultations held at both the ICMR and other national institutions with scientists, medical practitioners, lawyers, social scientists and activists.
- To ensure that ART clinics in India are accredited, regulated and supervised.
- Compulsory documentary evidence of the financial arrangement for surrogacy
- Involvement of ART bank in surrogate recruitment and their monetary aspects
- A known (relative) or unknown person to couple can act as a surrogate
- Maximum age limit to surrogate mother : 45years
- Maximum attempts as a surrogate: 3

2008: The Assisted Reproductive Technology (Regulation) Bill

- Establishment of National Advisory Board & State Boards
- ART procedures including surrogacy shall be available to all persons including single persons, married couples and unmarried couples.
- Legally enforceable surrogacy agreement
- Age limit for surrogate mother : 21 to 45 years
- No surrogate mother shall undergo embryo transfer more than three times for the same couple.
- The birth certificate issued in respect of a baby born through surrogacy shall bear the name(s) of the genetic parents / parent of the baby
- The person or persons who have availed of the services of a surrogate mother shall be legally bound to accept the custody of the child / children irrespective of any abnormality that the child / children may have, and the refusal to do so shall constitute an offence

- Foreigners, OCI, NRI, PIO are allowed to seek surrogacy by appointing responsible local guardian and providing documentation to the clinic that they will be able to take child born outside India to their country.

2010: The Assisted Reproductive Technology (Regulation) Bill

- Age limit for Surrogate Mother: 21 to 35 years
- Not more than 5 successive live births in surrogate mothers including her own children
- Only Indian citizens shall have a right to act as a surrogate, and no ART bank/ART clinics shall receive or send an Indian for surrogacy abroad.
- For foreigners, OCI, NRI, PIO seeking surrogacy in India along with local guardians following documentation is must.
- A letter from either the embassy of the Country in India or from the foreign ministry of the Country, clearly and unambiguously stating that (a) the country permits surrogacy, and (b) the child born through surrogacy in India, will be permitted entry in the Country as a biological child of the commissioning couple/individual
- If the foreign party seeking surrogacy fails to take delivery of the child born to the surrogate mother, the local guardian shall be legally obliged to take delivery of the child and be free to hand the child over to an adoption agency, if the commissioned party or their legal representative fails to claim the child within one months of the birth of the child.
- In case of adoption or the legal guardian having to bring up the child, the child will be given Indian citizenship.

2014: The Assisted Reproductive Technology (Regulation) Bill

- To establish the National Advisory Board, the State Advisory Boards and the National Registry for the accreditation, regulation and supervision of ART clinics and the ART banks, for prevention of misuse of ART including surrogacy, for safe and ethical practice of ART services

- Appropriate formula and mechanism shall be developed under Rules for payment of compensation to the surrogate mother and to transfer the funds to the bank account of the surrogate mother at different stages starting from signing of the agreement till the child/children is/are handed over to the commissioning parents.
- If there are any complications that have arisen during pregnancy (i.e. Gestational Diabetes, Chronic Hypertension etc.) which are likely to continue for the rest of the life of surrogate mother then it shall be covered appropriately under insurance.
- Age limit for surrogate mother : 23 years to 35 years
- Surrogate mother shall have at least one live child of her own with minimum age of three years.
- No woman shall act as a surrogate for more than one successful live birth in her life and with not less than two years interval between two deliveries.
- Surrogate mother shall be subjected to maximum three cycles of medications .
- Surrogacy for foreigners in India shall not be allowed.
- The spouse of the surrogate mother shall certify in his written consent that he will take care of the well being of the existing child/children of their own specially during the surrogacy agreement period and till his wife who is acting as a surrogate mother is free from the obligation of agreement.
- An Overseas Citizen of India (OCIs), People of Indian Origin (PIOs) and foreigner married to an Indian citizen, commissioning surrogacy in India shall –
    a. Be married and the marriage should have sustained at least for two years
    b. Use at least one gamete of their own in creation of the embryos
    c. Submit a certificate conveying that the woman is unable to conceive their own child and the certificate shall be attested by the appropriate government authority of that country.
    d. Obtain the requisite prior permission from the Foreigners Regional Registration Officer/Foreigners Registration Officer concerned for commissioning surrogacy

e. Have to come on a 'Medical Visa for surrogacy (MED-S) when they come to India for commissioning surrogacy
f. Appoint a local guardian
g. Insure the child or children born through the surrogacy, at the time of signing the agreement, till the age of twenty-one years or till the time of custody of the child or children is taken through appropriate Insurance Policy like JeevanBalya, whichever is earlier, for wellbeing and maintenance of the child or children
h. Require an 'exit' permission from the FRRO/FRO concerned for the child or children born through surrogacy before leaving India
i. A copy of the Birth Certificate(s) of the surrogate child/children will be retained by the Foreigners Regional Registration Officer/ Foreigners Registration Officer along with photocopies of the passport and cards of OCI, PIO, NRI & foreigners married to Indian citizens.

2016 : Surrogacy Bill

- Only Indian couples, who have been married for at least 5 years can opt for surrogacy, provided at least one of them have been proven to have fertility-related issues
- Only close relatives, not necessarily related by blood, will be able to offer altruistic surrogacy to the eligible couples.
- Commercial surrogacy is completely banned.
- It also bans unmarried people, live-in couples and homosexuals from opting for altruistic surrogacy. Now, foreigners, even Overseas Indians, cannot commission surrogacy.
- Surrogacy clinics will be allowed to charge for the services rendered in the course of surrogacy, but the surrogate mother cannot be paid, although payment can be made towards medical expenses only.
- The clinics will have to maintain records of surrogacy for 25 years.
- Commercial surrogacy, abandoning the surrogate child, exploitation of surrogate mother, selling/import of human embryo have all been categorized as violations that are punishable by a jail term of at least 10 years and a fine of up to Rs 10 lakh.

Chapter 6

The Surrogacy Bill 2016 – Treatment Becomes Crime

Since 2008, sporadic incidents at regular intervals involving surrogacy clearly demanded regulating this treatment. This law was in the making for almost a decade and was expected soon. The intended parents, the surrogate mothers, the legal authorities and the medical experts involved in surrogacy were looking forward to carefully designed regulations to avoid any kind of heartbreak to anyone. The ICMR guidelines were updated regularly over the years and had taken a final shape in 2014.

On 24th August 2016 the Union Cabinet passed the Surrogacy Bill 2016, which took everyone by surprise. This was not actually expected- A total ban on commercial surrogacy. A total ban on commercial surrogacy. It clearly reflected the exhaustion of the government on this issue. Surrogacy could not be allowed to continue as it is.

Most people still cannot believe the draconian nature of this bill. It clearly reflected the exhaustion of the government on this issue. For some reason, surrogacy could not be allowed to continue as it is.

The Provisions of the Surrogacy Bill 2016 are as Follows

Ban on Commercial Surrogacy, Only Altruistic Surrogacy Allowed that too by a Close Relative

This is an understandable reaction from the government, because there are many to talk against commercial surrogacy, but very few to defend. If a poor woman will be exploited, then it cannot be allowed. The altruistic concept of carrying a baby for someone else is allowed in the bill as long as there was no exchange of money beyond the medical bills. In addition, this altruistic form of surrogacy can only be done with the help of a close relative.

This close relative should be married and have her own child. It will be almost impossible for an infertile couple to find this close relative to carry their pregnancy and that too for no money. In this modern age, people are busy in their own lives. This has led to the breakup of the joint families and resulted in nuclear families. Women in this modern age are now very aggressive about their education and careers. They are themselves thinking of not having their own children, let alone carrying for others. It will be difficult for the couple to even ask for such help and even if the close relative agrees, the couple will feel miserable to have their child out of sympathy from a relative. This obligation can act on their mind for their lifetime. In this case, the couple will find a close relative from the rural connections. In this part of India, there is a still a lot of conservative mindset. The young lady may wish to help even, but her husband and his family may have objections for this. This may lead to friction in her family and can complicate her life. Under these circumstances, various practices may happen. The treatment may go underground. Couples may tempt the seniors in the poor family of a close relative to accept this treatment, but unofficially. The recently unveiled kidney racket in Mumbai is evidence that underground practices can start. This will put the lives of the young women at risk. In some cases, there can be coercion by the family of the intended parents to forcibly do surrogacy for them. Is it possible that the sperms from the husband are just put in the vagina of the close relative and she conceives without IVF treatment? This becomes traditional surrogacy with genetic link to the close relative and leads to maternal bonding. This has a high chance of genetic abnormality in the resulting baby, because it is like consanguinity.

One of the main reasons for couples to prefer the current format of commercial surrogacy is that they can keep it hidden from everyone, if they wish to do so. They may choose to keep it this way and not disclose this to their child. This is a very individual thing and it is best left for the couple to decide how they wish to handle the family and the society. In the altruistic form of surrogacy, especially when they use donor eggs and in the case of adoption, the couple cannot keep this hidden. It is open for the whole world to know as to what was done. What happens when this child faces the birth mother regularly. How does the child react to having two mothers, the genetic and the birth mother? Which way will the child's feelings go? Our society is not yet ready to accept these situations in a positive spirit. A woman or a couple who is unable to bear a child is still considered inferior and faces isolation. The reason most couples wish to keep their modes of treatment hidden is not because they are ashamed, but because they will face humiliation by family, friends and the relatives. They will have no control on the fallouts of this open secret. They fear that the child may face the same level of humiliation in events, in school, amongst friends and this is why they wish to protect their child by not disclosing the details of the treatment that was undertaken. It is very easy to advise people to adopt and to do surrogacy using their close relatives, but it is very tough for them to face the society and live a normal life. It is not the couple who wants to hide or not adopt. It is our very own society who have their own children who become very judgmental and make their lives miserable. The law is necessary to control the society, but if the culture and traditions are so heavily embedded in the minds of the people, which law can penetrate deep. It will need many more years for our people to change their thinking. They need education and awareness on the subject.

We are facing the same attitude in the case of the girl child. Our traditions and culture and the bias against girls in every sense is the roadblock. Any draconian law, any actions against the doctors is like giving medications to reduce fever, but the underlying infection has not been cured. In time, the fever will not respond to the medications and the infection will kill the person. These problems are so deep rooted, going on from our ancient times. Where do you start? It will take few lifetimes to make a small change.

As mentioned earlier in this book, the current form of surrogacy should be given the Altruistic status, because the money paid to the surrogate mother does not make it truly commercial. The surrogate mother has good intentions to help the couple and at the same time she wants to help her children and family. The money paid should be considered fair compensation for her time, effort, loss of earnings, fees for arranging help at home, the health coverage and so on. The compensation can be decided by the government and payments can be monitored.

This form should be called as "Altruistic compensatory Surrogacy."

One of the main contentions with the current form of surrogacy is that it is exploitative in nature. The bill may stop the exploitation in the current format, but it will lead to other exploitation of these women, which we will never even know.

"It is equivalent to say to a person who is vomiting to stop drinking water. At the same time, the persons body needs water. If this is not given as intravenous fluids, the person will anyways die. With vomiting, at least some amount of fluid was available to the body. The best thing is to treat the cause of vomiting so that all the fluid reaches the right place and the person benefits."

In the process of banning surrogacy for the rare issues that arose in the past, we will deprive thousands of deserving couples from the joy of parenthood that comes with surrogacy. This law is not about the doctors it is about the citizens of this country who are suffering silently and who do not have a voice. We must be sensitive to their needs. They very well deserve this.

Who can do Altruistic Surrogacy?

a) Only Indian couples are allowed to do surrogacy.

b) The couple should be married for 5 years and should have proven infertility.

c) Foreigners, NRIs, OCI and PIO card holders cannot undertake surrogacy in India. One of the reasons cited for this provision is that this group has higher divorce rates. In other words, the rights of the unborn child are also to be considered.

d) The couple should not have any children from before, from this marriage or even any previous marriage. The logic is that there can be discrimination between the children, maybe at the time of property distribution. It is assumed that real brothers and sisters do not have property disputes and even if that happens, it becomes acceptable.

If this is true, divorced men and women cannot be allowed to remarry, because step brothers and sisters can also face this problem of discrimination.

e) Couples with abnormal children can go for surrogacy. This implies that we consider them disadvantaged and we assume that they are unhappy. Life is an experience. This couple have a different form of experience. By no means this can be considered any less than that of the others. Just in case if this couple does go for surrogacy in pursuit of a "normal" child, what happens about the discrimination. Can there be discrimination between the two? Can it lead to sibling jealousy?

The National Regulator: All stake holders involved in surrogacy welcome this part of the bill. This body will oversee the clinics and hospitals offering surrogacy treatment. This is what exactly everyone wants- Regulations and Regulator. Unfortunately, banning commercial surrogacy and allowing altruistic surrogacy will not leave much for the regulator to oversee, because even if it happens, it will be hidden under covers. Instead, make it open and regulate. You can at least see what is happening and what needs to be done.

Legal aid to surrogate mothers: This is also not much required for altruistic surrogacy done within close relatives of the family. There will be no room for legal actions within the family, because it can have serious implications for the entire families well-being.

The punishment:

- The intended parents have to accept the child born out of surrogacy. If not they can face a jail penalty.
- In a similar manner, the surrogate mother should be expected to follow the medical instructions and care for the pregnancy. This makes it fair for both parties.
- Anyone doing commercial surrogacy will face Rupees 10 lakhs as fine and 10 years in jail. It appears that all governments believe that doctors are the culprit example- PCPNDT and now the Surrogacy bill. It is the mindset of the people, which is responsible for the social issues. It is our culture and the traditions that have to be blamed. Punishing doctors and declaring 10 year jail terms just to terrorize the medical profession is bad for the profession. India has very few doctors and our challenges are huge. The profession is probably at its all time low feeling. Most doctors would not want their children to take up this profession. It is a bad sign. Many wish to leave the country to practice abroad. Arresting doctors for clerical errors as in PCPNDT is sending very wrong signals across the medical community. Smaller hospitals and Nursing homes are up against the challenges posed by corporate hospitals, government regulations, people expectations, public bashing, insurance companies and the ever increasing costs of running hospitals. This will eventually lead to closure of the friendly doctor in the neighborhood and the healthcare will become a disaster as in the UK and the USA.

We have the best doctors in the world even after so many have left the country. This has made us the number 1 destination in the world for medical tourism and number 3 in the world in the quality of medical facilities and services. At the same time, we are 97th in the world in the hunger index, one out of every twenty children die before the age of 5 and we have one of the worst child mortality rates in the world. We need a lot of doctors and we need them to work enthusiastically.

In other countries, surrogacy is either outlawed altogether or regulated through legal instruments to ensure a fair deal for all the parties involved. In Italy, Finland and Iceland, it is banned altogether. In others, like UK and New Zealand, only commercial surrogacy is banned. Altruistic surrogacy – meaning where the surrogate mother is not paid but carries the child out of love or compassion – is allowed.

In Israel, Ukraine and Russia, surrogacy is allowed but regulated by the government to protect the rights of both the commissioning parent or parents and the surrogate mother. In the US, different states have different laws, but it is generally quite easy for prospective parents to have children through surrogacy.

Questions Raised by the Surrogacy Bill

Do we believe that couples with an abnormal child are less happier than those with normal children?

What if the couple cannot find a close relative to do surrogacy for them?

What if the couple takes a divorce if the close relative is pregnant?

Does the couple have right to their own privacy about their reproduction, because with close relative surrogacy the treatment will be out in the open?

What happens if the close relative feels attached to the child at a later stage?

What happens when the child calls the close relative "Mummy?"

How would the child handle two mothers – birth mother and the legal mother?

What if the birth mother (close relative) wishes to take back the child if anything happens to her children?

Can this lead to a divorce of the close relative if she does surrogacy against the wishes of her husband and inlaws?

Can a couple put the sperms of the husband in the vagina of the close relative so that the pregnancy can result without IVF treatment and also they get known eggs. In this case, there is a risk of abnormality in the child due to consanguinity?

What if the couple does not feel comfortable to adopt?

Is it wrong to want your own genes in your own child?

Can adoption be forced upon anyone ?

If surrogacy is unsafe and inappropriate for foreigners and single individuals, should adoption be allowed for them?

Is it not insulting to the couples who have tried for years to have a baby and finally chosen to do surrogacy to be blamed of doing it for fashion?

Why does a couple have to be married for 5 years, if the lady has a serious health issue or does not have a womb for any reason?

What happens if a woman has a hysterectomy (removal of the womb) for reasons such as bleeding during delivery, cancer, fibroids and other gynaecological reasons?

Does a woman have the right over her reproduction?

Can she decide to carry a baby for another couple for her personal reasons?

Is it wrong to charge a fee for the time, effort and loss of earnings for a period of almost a year?

Is it wrong to compensate the surrogate mother for her loss of earnings, expenses, time, effort and medical fees?

Carrying a baby by a close relative can be done under pressure. Why should this be allowed?

Why only close relative can do altruism?

Should a surrogate mother be proud or ashamed?

Will a needy woman get exploited in bar dancing, sex working, as cooks, housemaids?

Surrogacy treatment will help the infertile couples, the surrogate mothers, the nation and even charity can benefit if this is all put together in a good framework?

Can we have a law to arrest people if they harass infertile couples?

Can this ban make surrogacy treatment go underground?

Can the close relative get paid internally and the treatment gets called altruistic?

Will the close family members of the close relative object to such treatment?

Can a family force the daughter in law to carry a pregnancy for someone in the family. Is she in a position to refuse such a request?

Is it right that a couple with years of suffering and prolonged treatment has to depend upon the sympathy of a close relative to have their family?

Chapter 7

Surrogacy is a treatment. Adoption is a choice

Surrogacy is a medical option. Adoption is a social option. It is natural human tendency to want a genetic link to the child.

This is a choice which some people have to make at some stage of their treatment. Both options are always offered to the couples **(Chart 12)**. Most couples are actually unaware of the details about surrogacy even at this advanced stage of their treatment. They have never needed to educate themselves about this option. At this stage, their deep desire to have their genetic link to the baby overrides and in most cases they prefer surrogacy. There is a growing number of couples who are not wanting even their own children. It is generally tough for them to accept the option of adoption. Some have even registered for adoption, but they are unsure and change their mind. Many couples wanting to adopt have been very disappointed with the procedure for adopting a child.

Almost all in this situation prefer surrogacy over adoption for reasons such as:

1) Surrogacy gives them the option of keeping their treatment confidential, whereas in adoption they are not in control and everyone comes to know about it

2) In surrogacy, they may choose to not disclose the method of conception to the child, but in adoption this is almost impossible

3) The social disclosure in adoption makes it very difficult for the couple to protect themselves and the child from the isolation and gossip from family, friends and relatives. This happens due to the orthodox

conservative kind of thought process, which is deep-rooted in the society still.

4) Conception with the help of technology is even still not fully understood and accepted. Let alone, further advanced options such as egg donation, surrogacy and adoption.

5) Adoption is a very tedious and time consuming process. Some couples have tried this route and got back to their own treatment, because they were very unhappy with the process of adoption.

6) In adoption, they have the fear that the adopted child may not settle and their may be emotional issues. In this case, the agencies can even take back the child after few months. These are the fears expressed by the couples who have entered the adoption process and then withdrawn.

7) There is a long waiting time for the adoption to happen.

Some couples willingly accept adoption and have been successful. Almost all of them feel happy, but some of them still think of their own child, because our society is still unwilling to accept the adopted child. Intentionally or unintentionally, the family, friends and relatives tend to hurt the couple and the child. This can make it very difficult for the settled family to regroup themselves. The couple need s a letter from the treating doctor to certify that the couple cannot achieve a pregnancy of their own and are justified in thinking of an adoption.

Chart 12: Surrogacy vs Adoption

Surrogacy	Adoption
Genetic link to the baby	No genetic link
Controlled process	Uncertainty
Uniform guidelines	No uniform common stature to govern adoption law. Laws are different for different religion.
Organized process	Difficult, intricate & time consuming process
No parental right of surrogate mother on child.	Birth mother can change her mind & can discontinue her adoption plan. She may want to maintain post adoption relationship with child.
Till now, there was no age limit for intended parents	Age limit for adoptive parents
Can be kept confidential	Open to the society
Easier for emotional bonding	The child may find it difficult to adapt to the new home
New Bill does not allow foreigners, NRIs and the OCI card holders to do surrogacy	The government regulations allow foreigners, NRIs and the OCI card holders to adopt
Single parents and divorced are not allowed Surrogacy	Single parents and divorced individuals can dopt
People with previous children cannot do Surrogacy	People with porevious children upto 4 in number can adopt

Some adopt voluntarily and that is also good. They have a different way of looking at life. Their upbringing, their experience of life and their views are very individual and that must be respected too. But, those views cannot be forced on others, because each person is living life in his or her own way and likes to have the freedom to do so.

In some cases, couples prefer to take embryo adoption. In this treatment, the couple may have gone through many years of fertility treatment. Instead of going for surrogacy or adoption, they make take embryo adoption. In this treatment, the eggs and the sperms are borrowed and an embryo created using IVF technology and transferred back to the wife. She carries the pregnancy and does the delivery without anyone realizing the nature of the underlying process. This is sometimes given preference over surrogacy or adoption, because the couple is able to maintain their confidentiality. They are able to start a family life without anyone's involvement. Once the couple is in terms with this arrangement, they are very happy with the baby and they do not have worry about explaining the treatment process to anyone.

Chapter 8

The World is more Commercial than Altruistic

India is named as the "Surrogacy capital of the world," but Nobody wants to call India "The medical tourism capital of the world"

Each country decides their own laws on the basis of their requirements **(Chart 13)**. When the countries of the world are divided on their position in the matter of surrogacy and when there are different forms of surrogacy that are acceptable and unacceptable, it is clear that it is not about being right or wrong. It is open to your own interpretation depending on what is suitable in your own country. In some countries altruistic surrogacy is allowed and some even allow commercial surrogacy. In some European countries, sex working has been legalized and they also have full constitutional rights. Some countries have death penalty and some do not. A law in some country may be completely unacceptable to the people of another country, but they may be fine with it. It is not necessary that each country handles each issue similarly, because there are too many variables that change from place to place. If the surrogacy agreement can be made legally enforceable, then it becomes easy for the country to allow the treatment. Each country decides whether they recognize the birth mother or the biological mother as the legal mother. Once these uncertainties are defined, it becomes much easier to define your position in this matter and the further rules and regulations and the necessary penalties just follow.

It is very inappropriate for the westerners to criticize the law of this country. People in the west have been giving names to surrogacy such as rent a womb, baby farming and so on. According to them motherhood is shameful if this is achieved with the help of another person. If the government can regulate this treatment and stand in pride to defend the interests of our people, the negative criticism will stop. If commercial surrogacy is illegal in the UK, Australia or Canada, they may have their own reasons. The women there may be charging a lot of money and maybe they have numerous legal issues that may be happening in their country. They may not have so much importance for parenthood. Infertility may not be so much a stigma in those countries as in India. Our infertile couples may be facing bigger challenges in the society than their people. In some states of America, commercial surrogacy is legal and they would not be affected by what laws are made in other countries.

It is obvious that the altruistic surrogacy program has failed worldwide, because as soon as India was able to offer the quality care to the world, their patients came flocking to India for treatment. If the altruistic surrogacy program was successful outside India, why would foreigners come to India for treatment. They all came here, had children and went home with gratitude and fond memories for their lifetime. India had made a special place in their lives. They even started coming back to India for further treatment. This successful program had opened up so many opportunities that helped our people. The westerners could not bear this benefit to India and so gave bad names to this treatment. The world would be quick to call India the "Surrogacy Capital of The world" or the "Surrogacy hub of the world." You will not hear them call us "The Medical Tourism Capital of the world" or "The Medical Tourism hub of the world." There is an element of jealousy when the world sees India flourish in anything. There was some justification in their allegations about exploitation, but these were our internal matters and our government was looking into the issues and we were about to have good regulations. After this, the treatment would have become a win-win situation for all.

In time, when the economical conditions would change and our women would have other opportunities and research would provide other options to help our infertile couples, the nature of this treatment would automatically change.

Chart 13: Surrogacy Laws by Country

S. No	Country	Commercial Surrogacy	Altruistic Surrogacy
1	India	Allowed	Allowed
2	US California, Arkansas, New Hampshire	Allowed	Allowed
3	Israel "State Controlled Surrogacy" – First Country in the world	Allowed	Allowed
4	Russia	Allowed	Allowed
5	Greece	Allowed	Allowed
6	Ukraine	Allowed	Allowed
7	Georgia	Allowed	Allowed
8	Thailand	Not Allowed	Allowed
9	UK	Not Allowed	Allowed
10	US New York	Not Allowed	Allowed
11	Australia	Not Allowed	Allowed
12	Canada	Not Allowed	Allowed
13	Hong Kong	Not Allowed	Allowed
14	Belgium	Not Allowed	Allowed
15	Netherlands	Not Allowed	Allowed
16	Hungary	Not Allowed	Allowed
17	New Zealand	Not Allowed	Allowed
18	Portugal	Not Allowed	Allowed
19	South Africa	Not Allowed	Allowed
20	US Michigan	Not Allowed	Not Allowed
21	Spain	Not Allowed	Not Allowed
22	Italy	Not Allowed	Not Allowed
23	Iceland	Not Allowed	Not Allowed

Chapter 9

Surrogacy – The Media and the Peoples Opinion

It is very clear from the following survey carried out amongst the intended parents and the surrogate mothers that they wish to have regulation and not ban on the surrogacy treatment **(Chart 14)**. There is strong message that this group of people to whom the law will affect are unhappy, but at the same time unable to voice their feelings. The societal pressures have choked them. They will express their feelings when you speak with them, but almost all want secrecy as if they have done some crime. They know that they should be able to come out in the open with pride, but the society is still not mature enough to understand their pain and suffering. They feel that they will not be able to lead a normal life, if they disclose their involvement in this treatment.

Chart 14: Statistical Survey Done in 30 Cases of Surrogacy Treatment

Intended Parent Survey	
Average age of women to be Intended Parent via surrogacy	40 years (29 to 54 years)
Average age of men to be Intended Parent via surrogacy	42 years (32 to 58 years)
Average duration of marriage before doing surrogacy	12 years (3 to 30 years)
Should Commercial surrogacy be banned	Yes-0%
Should Commercial Surrogacy get regulated	Yes-100%
Surrogate mother survey	
Should Commercial surrogacy be banned	Yes-0%
Should Commercial Surrogacy get regulated	Yes-100%

The Indian Express Unequal by law

We need effective, non-discriminatory regulation of surrogacy. Draft bill is biased, exclusionary

ANALYSIS

Surrogacy Bill's missteps
BY AMRITA PANDE
12 SEPTEMBER 2016

Is the prohibitory approach, adopted by the Surrogacy (Regulation) Bill 2016, really the best way to protect the rights of surrogates and their children in India?

Gulf News – 24 Sept 2016

Surrogacy bill stirs womb trade row

Draft law bars foreigners, single people and married couples with children from opting for surrogate births

Image Credit: AFP

September 23, 2016

News 18 31st August 2016

After Surrogacy Bill Creates a Storm, ModiGovt Could Change Some Provisions

The surrogacy bill is dangerous overreach

Ideological bias has trumped economic and ethical logic

Livemint 31st August 2016

Dr. Sandeep Mane

New surrogacy Bill bars married couples with kids, NRIs, gays, live-ins, foreigners

The government on Wednesday approved a bill that bans commercial surrogacy, and bars single people, married couples who have biological/adopted children, live-in partners and homosexuals from opting for surrogacy.

By: Express News Service August 25, 2016

External Affairs Minister SushmaSwaraj said foreigners, NRIs and PIOs who hold Overseas Citizens of India cards have been barred from opting for surrogacy as "divorces are very common in foreign countries." (Express File Photo by PremNath Pandey)

F. INDIA

Surrogacy Bill 2016 imposes unjust bans and does not focus on the real issues

Gita Aravamudan Aug 28, 2016

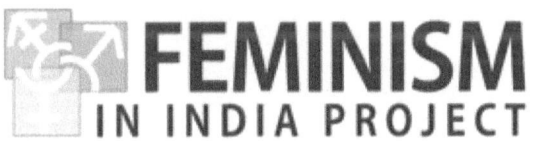

A Critical Analysis Of The Surrogacy Regulation Bill 2016

by MALAVIKA RAVI

— August 31, 2016

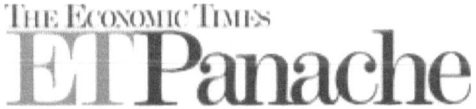

Banning commercial surrogacy will expose women to exploitation

Aug 28, 2016

By Hari G Ramasubramanian

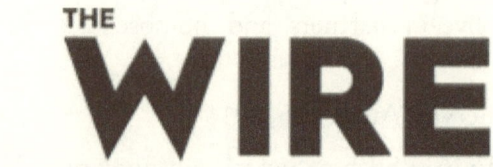

Where Does the Surrogacy Bill Stand on the Rights of the Surrogate?
BY PARIJATA BHARDWAJ ON 31/08/2016

The Diplomat

Image Credit: Pixabay/Unsplash

India Must Tread Cautiously on Surrogacy Law

India's new surrogacy bill attempts to legislate morality, while the women at risk may not see benefits.

By Anuradha Sharma

August 31, 2016

IMPORTANT

All that is wrong with the new surrogacy bill

IMAGE: Shah Rukh Khan with son Abram, who was born through a surrogate. The proposed bill would not allow such a procedure.

As a mother, as a woman, as a human being, Savera R Someshwar/Rediff.com is horrified by some of the provisions of the Surrogacy Regulation Bill, 2016.

Supermom of State, SushmaSwaraj, gifts India a Sanskari Surrogacy Bill

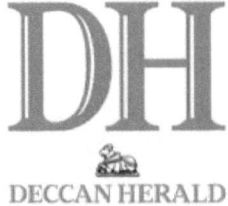

Thursday 01 September 2016
Surrogacy bill regressive, preachy

Thursday, September 01, 2016

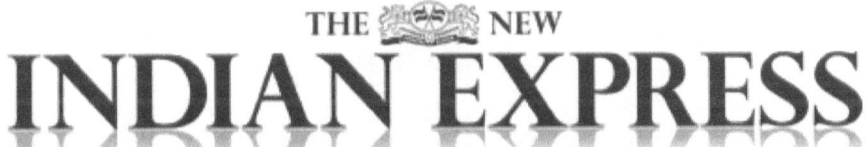

Devil is in the detail in surrogacy bill

By Express News Service nie

Published: 27th August 2016

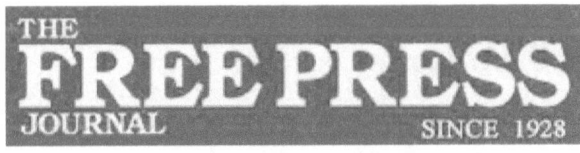

From liberal democracy to nanny state with surrogacy bill

— By Bhavdeep Kang | Aug 31, 2016

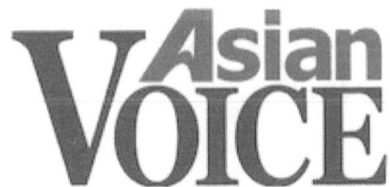

Surrogacy Bill: Fight between Rights and Morality
Wednesday 31ˢᵗ August 2016

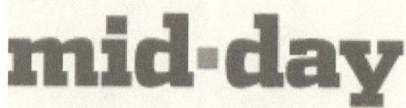

Amit Karkhanis: Proposed surrogacy bill is a demon in the making

By Amit Karkhanis | Posted 26-Aug-2016

It is unfortunate that the government has missed a historical opportunity to regularise the surrogacy industry and has made it rather regressive and backward

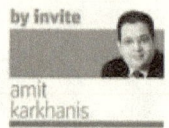

Last Modified: Thu, Sep 01 2016

The surrogacy bill gets it all wrong

Bans create black markets and greater vulnerability, and take away an economic option from working-class women

Vrinda Marwah

Surrogacy bill bother for parents

TNN | Updated: Oct 6, 2016

Some articles in support of the Bill:

THE HINDU

Why the Surrogacy Bill is necessary
SOUMYA SWAMINATHAN

HINDUSTAN TIMES
The new surrogacy bill will stop exploitation of women

Hindustan Times

Updated: Aug 25, 2016

Chapter 10

Surrogacy Solution – Please Heal it Not Kill

Surrogacy is currently a choice that desperate couples make when they are unable to conceive. It is also a matter of choice that the surrogate mother makes willingly in her given personal situation. The couple accepts this as a treatment option to fulfill their dream and the surrogate mother accepts this to fulfill her requirement and to help the couple in the process. Uniquely, there is a blend of medical, legal, social, financial, moral, ethical, constitutional, parental, emotional and international issues involved in surrogacy. Lack of regulation and a suitable law has made it difficult to control some of the issues. It is amazing that the treatment has done so well inspite of the total freedom that it had. Rare diversions from the norm and occasional international complications brought disrepute to the treatment. It has been a life-changer for thousands of Indian and International couples.

One thing is certain and everyone agrees, that it needs to be regulated and should not be allowed to continue in its current format. The debate is whether surrogacy needs a commercial regulation or an altruistic form or a total ban. Surrogacy is an option available to the surrogate mothers to help their children and their family. Will there be an exploitation of these women, because they are helpless and desperate? It is hard to believe that this will never happen. The next question is whether any exploitation can be prevented. If all issues are brought out in the open, there will be no scope for exploitation. The surrogate mothers must get good treatment and no one must be allowed to cheat them. At the same time, there should be clear terms defined so that the interests of the intended parents can also be safeguarded.

Regulate or Ban?

Regulation would involve creating a platform which should ensure that there are minimal risks to the surrogate mothers and the intended parents. It should check that the middlemen do not misuse the surrogacy arrangement for their personal gains. This would be admittedly tough to achieve, but does this justify banning commercial surrogacy? There are numerous examples where regulation is tough, but ban cannot be the solution. PCPNDT Act aims to regulate the use of ultrasound scans to avoid sex determination. Banning sonography technology will totally eradicate the issue, but that cannot be the solution. The Medical Termination of Pregnancy (MTP) Act aims to regulate the choice of termination of pregnancy. Banning MTP cannot be the solution. But then what about smoking, which kills. Can there be any justification to not ban smoking.

This leads us to ask the question **is carrying a pregnancy for someone else morally correct**? The answer is that having a child through surrogacy is not a luxury for the couple, it is their basic purpose to live. At the same time it is enabling the surrogate mother to help her children and her family. Hence, the moral standing of the surrogacy treatment cannot be questioned, because this is done by choice, without any coercion and with positive intentions.

So the next question is **whether it is ethically correct to pay money to carry a pregnancy** for someone else? It is understood that payment in receipt of service qualifies to be called commercial, but does the quantity of the payment matter? Is it wrong for the surrogate mother to get compensated for her time, loss of earnings, efforts, expenses, health fees. Does the recovery of her expenses make it a profit-making commercial act. Lets take the example of charitable organizations, which are non-profit making. Does that mean that charitable institutions cannot expect a nominal fee to cover their costs. Almost all charitable institutions charge fees. It is well known that charitable hospital trusts charge regular fees to patients. Some trusts are very rich, but that does not make them commercial. They are still given the tax benefits. Why??- Because there intentions are to help someone. In the process they are not exploiting their customers to make profit. The profit that they make is made useful for social uplifting. In a similar manner, the surrogate mothers are covering their costs and in this way they are uplifting the lives of their children and their family. The intended parents who pay for their services are not just the rich people. They make their arrangements to raise the required money and take the help of the surrogate mothers only as a last option. In a similar manner, those who can have their treatment in themselves and those who can have their own children will not do surrogacy. Inability to have their own children should be the criteria for surrogacy. The reasons for this inability can be medical in majority of the cases and social in some. Our society is very harsh on the couples who are unable to have their children naturally. This is why the intended parents and the surrogate mothers try to keep the good work hidden. Most of them wish to keep their identity hidden. This is very unfortunate. The government must give it the full framework for good recognition of these citizens. They deserve respect and not humiliation. Infertile couples must be protected from the ill treatment given to them by the society. If this can be done, maybe some more couples can be encouraged to adopt a child. Adopting a child will become more acceptable if the society's views can be changed. It cannot be forced on to people, especially when the society is not yet so welcoming for this. If the attempts at regulation fail, then ban will become necessary as the last option. A well-planned regulatory mechanism will almost certainly avoid a ban on surrogacy.

How to REGULATE

The ART Guidelines of 2014 have very well outlined the structure for the ART Regulatory framework. The same has been followed below with minor variations.

Surrogacy can be regulated by two steps:

1 Legally Enforceable Surrogacy Agreement and

2 Stringent Regulatory Mechanism

Legally Enforceable Surrogacy Agreement:

Surrogacy agreements that are legally enforceable should be carefully drafted so that all issues relating to malpractices, mal-intentions and exploitation can be prevented. The payment structure should be clearly outlined so that there are no financial irregularities. The terms and conditions for the surrogate mothers, the intended parents and the medical experts should be clearly outlined.

Duties of the surrogate mother:

- The agreement should define the eligibility to become a surrogate mother
- She maintains herself in good health and follows the medical instructions given
- She fulfills her commitment as outlined in the agreement. This involves, taking adequate rest, timely medicines, performing the tests as required for the normal continuation of the pregnancy

Duties of the intended parents:

- They must not make any demands that may be detrimental to the health of the surrogate mother
- They must not expect the surrogate mother to do anything against her religious belief
- They must accept the opinion of the treating medical expert
- They will not refuse to accept the child born out of the surrogacy. If they do so, then this may attract a jail term. This is applicable even if the child is abnormal or of an unwanted sex.
- They must fulfill their financial commitments as per the agreed payment schedule
- There should be financial provisions for the surrogate child in case of divorce, death of the couple or any unwillingness to accept the child.
- They should nominate the guardian who must have defined duties and responsibilities to fulfill in case the parents of the surrogate child are unable or unwilling to fulfill their role.

The surrogate mother maintains her control over her body, but the intended parents maintain the control on the pregnancy. In case the interest of the surrogate mothers health and the well-being of the pregnancy clash, the medical experts advise will become important. Surrogacy must be governed by the MTP act, PNDT act and so on. The safety of the surrogate mother should be given the prime importance at all times. The surrogate mother will have the choice to stay at her own home if this is considered safe as per the medical advise. If she stays in the surrogate home, then all the appropriate facilities should be made available for her comfortable stay. She should be given hygienic living conditions and healthy diet during her pregnancy. All necessary medications must be made available to her as required. In case of any medical complications arising in the pregnancy, the surrogate mother will be given complete medical attention, even if it means admission to another hospital. The surrogate mother will not be burdened with the bills of such medical care given to her. The mode of delivery is decided by the treating doctor ensuring that the surrogate mother understands the decisions and has been consented properly. Post-delivery the surrogate mother will be given proper supplements for upto three months. In the rare event of the death of the surrogate mother during her pregnancy due to reasons relating to the pregnancy or her health condition, except accidental death, there would be a compensation in the form of an insurance that would be given to the family of the surrogate mother.

Chart 15: Mechanism to Regulate Surrogacy

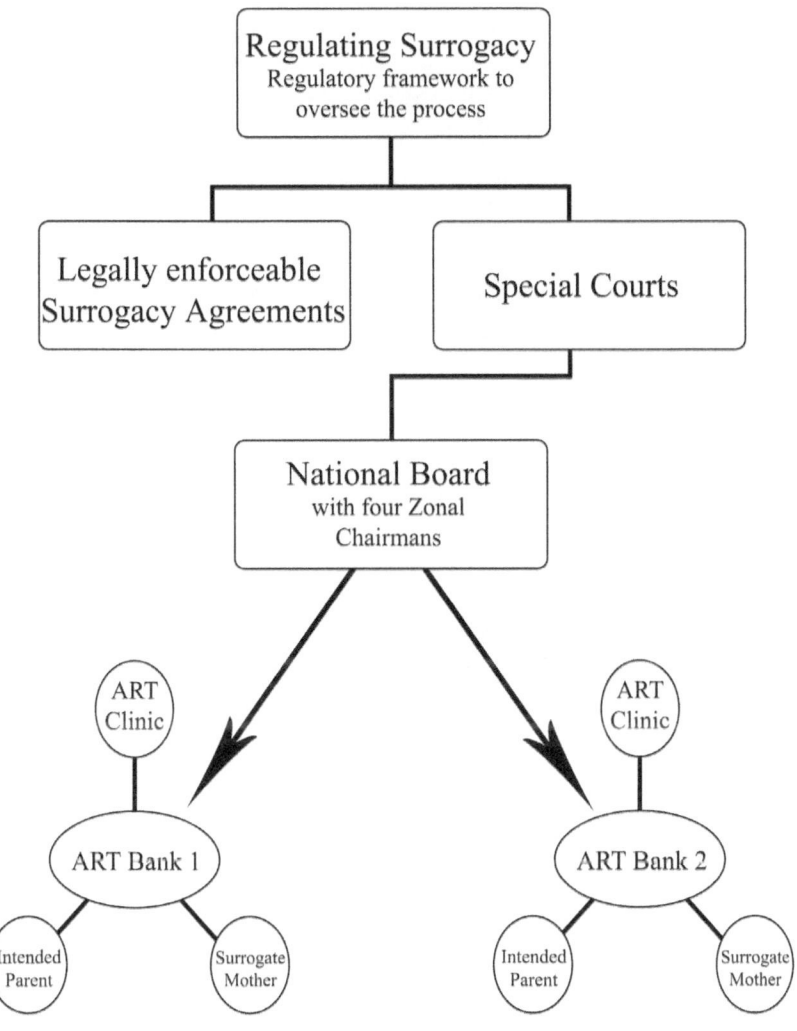

A) National Regulatory board:

This would be a national board to register and monitor the surrogacy practices in India. This would comprise of a group of individuals from different fields related to the surrogacy services. The country can be divided into the four zones with each having their zonal representative (Chairman) in the central board. Each zonal chairman will supervise the surrogacy services within their zone and report to the central board. They will implement the process of registering the clinics for surrogacy. They will ensure that the set criteria are met. They are the brains behind the surrogacy services in India. This body gives the vision to this program. They will execute their vision with the help of the Executive bodies, Assisted Reproduction Technology (ART) Banks. They will also make inspections of the clinics from time to time to ensure that all is well. The national board will also have an advisory cell that can assist the ART banks in any complicated cases. Such cases can be discussed in the board meetings and decisions given in stipulated time periods.

B) Assisted Reproduction Technology (ART) Banks:

These are independent organizations providing donor and surrogacy services to the Assisted Reproductive Technology (ART) Clinics. The donor and surrogacy related work, which includes selection, recruitment and coordination can be carried out by them. The medical experts of each clinic will submit their patient details to the ART Bank, which should ensure that they meet the set criteria required to offer the particular treatment. If in doubt, they should refer the case to the national board. The decision of the national board will be final.

Duties of the ART bank:

1. To select and recruit donors and surrogate mothers for the ART clinics
2. To ensure that the treatment being offered is meeting the set criteria
3. To maintain records of all treatments undertaken
4. To get PCPNDT Registration and to follow the PCPNDT Act
5. To run a surrogate home for needy surrogate mothers who may wish to stay.

6. To submit the details of each surrogacy treatment to the national board
7. The banks will ensure that all the surrogacy agreements are in order. This would include the following:
   - Triparty Agreement between the intended parents(IP), the surrogate mother and the ART clinic
   - Agreement between the IP and the ART Bank
   - Any other relevant agreements that may be felt necessary

These agreements will be legally registered and should cover issues such as financial, legal, procedural and other commitments between the different parties. These carefully drafted agreements will become legally enforceable and those in breach of this will face the punishment. Ultimately, the ART banks will liaise with the national board to pass on the details of each surrogacy case undertaken by them.

C) Assisted Reproductive Technology (ART) Clinic:

Clinics offering surrogacy service will have to register

- There should be eligibility criteria for the clinics to fulfill
- Provisions for domestic, medical and legal help to the surrogates must be ensured
- Government Registry to keep the records of all the surrogacy cases

Who can do surrogacy

- Criteria for the married couples
- Constitutional rights of individuals such as singles, gay couples and people with children
- International law- Rules for foreign patients

Who can be a surrogate mother

Age criteria

How many children, including her own

How many surrogacy attempts

Plea to the Government

The citizens of India understand the concerns expressed by you regarding the surrogacy practice in our country. It is accepted that this cannot continue further in the current manner. Any form of exploitation must be stopped. Utilization of any poor woman for the financial gains of any group must not not be allowed.

In doing so, there are mainly two groups that will get affected by any legislation in this matter:

Group 1: The Surrogate Mothers

Group 2: The intended Parents

Both these groups have no voice, because they are suffering and they cannot tell that to anyone. All that is said is only on their behalf. Surrogacy is a unique medical treatment, which has massive social implications, for both, the surrogate mothers and the intended parents. The legislation governing this will have impact on the generations of both these groups. For them, it is not fashion, it is almost about life and death. Both are dying on a daily basis and the treatment makes life changing difference to them.

It is a humble request to give an opportunity for this treatment to be done under stringent regulation. During the time that regulations will be tried, there will be newer research and the medical experts can find ways in which to help the intended couples. One such example is uterine transplant, which is just on the horizon. We will hope that the country does socioeconomic progress and our poor get better education and skills, which will empower them to fulfill the needs of their children and their families by other means. We may be able to offer social security to our citizens in the future. If the regulation fails and there is no choice, then the ban becomes inevitable, irrespective of whether science has progressed or not and whether the poor are independent or not. We can only hope and pray that good regulations and sincere intentions by all involved parties will see happy days for all the stake holders and the nation benefits in the process. The current form of Surrogacy has Altruistic nature, because the surrogate mother does it selflessly for her children and her family. Her fees only amount to the compensation of her time, effort, loss of earnings, out of pocket expenses, which cannot be called commercial (profit-making).

Mother India should take pride in giving motherhood to the people. The surrogate mother and the intended mother share a beautiful relationship bonded by a baby. We deplore people who insult motherhood by calling it names such as renting a womb, baby farming, baby factories and so on. The same people will not admire India for achieving excellence in medical tourism. We, in India, believe in the family concept and surrogacy is all about creating happy families. Each country is free to make its own laws, which suit its own people. If they want their people to benefit, we are happy to oblige, because we believe that happy individuals, happy families, happy societies, happy nations will lead to peace and harmony.

If you still believe that we must ban commercial surrogacy in India now, the debate will rest here and we will ask our patients to accept their loss.

Regulate or Ban, whichever serves human interests best, must happen (Chart 16)

Chart 16: The Journey of Surrogacy- Legalised, Regulate, Ban

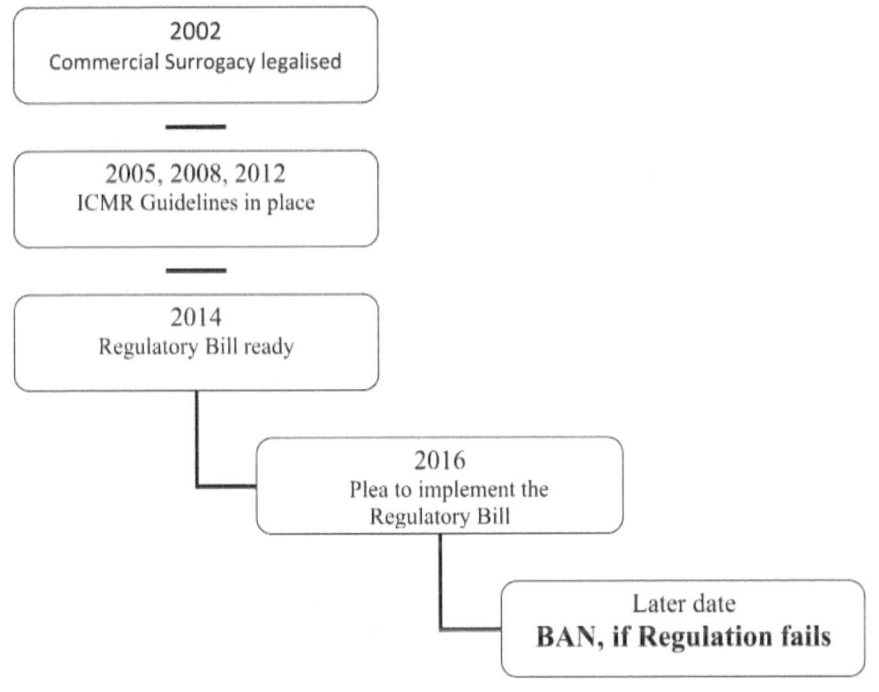

Chapter 11
FAQs-All Questions Must be Answered

1. **Like in the case of adoption, should the intended parents undertaking surrogacy not go through a stringent screening process**

   In the maximum number of cases the couples undertaking surrogacy have proven themselves to be a very commited couple. After 10 to 15 years of prolonged treatment, the couple cannot be doubted about their ability to provide the safe atmosphere to the unborn child). They do not need any further screening to prove that they deserve parenthood. In that case, should every desiring parent go through a screening test before producing their children.

2. **What about the rights of the unborn child in surrogacy?**

   The rights of the unborn child must certainly be protected. In the case of surrogacy, the rights of the unborn child will be very well protected if the regulations are made and followed. There are numerous other examples where the rights of the unborn child are not protected: a woman smoking or consuming alcohol in pregnancy, poor diet available during pregnancy.

3. **India is not short of children. Why do we need any more with surrogacy?**

   Having children is an individual need. We all come to live life as an experience. Each and every person deserves their share of experience, irrespective of your caste, creed, nationality, financial status

4. **India has many children abandoned by their biological parents. Why do we need artificial methods of reproduction like surrogacy**

   Having a child is an individual reproductive right. Children must not be abandoned in the first place. There should be serious punishment for those who abandon their children. If any couple voluntarily wishes to adopt, then it must be encouraged, but forcible adoption can be very dangerous. Science and technology is good if it helps to improve the quality of life. Assisted reproduction is like any other form of medical treatment and must continue to relieve the pain and suffering of an individual.

5. **As the surrogate mothers suffer exploitation, should surrogacy not be banned**

Exploitation of the surrogate mothers must not be allowed. But is banning a solution to their miseries. They may be saved from some instances of exploitation, but can they suffer even worse exploitation when they remain vulnerable. We must design a mechanism to protect them and ensure fairness.

6. **Surrogate mothers may have complications. Who will look after them?**

These are young women being managed by expert doctors with all the financial support. The IPs also have their interest in looking after the surrogate mother, because they are helping their baby in the process. The surrogate mothers life gets the first priority and then the pregnancy. The treating doctor has to ensure that the surrogate mothers health interests are taken care of at all times. The intended parents and the clinic should ensure that she is given the health support that she needs. Her health is of prime importance.

7. **Who will insure for the surrogate mother**

The surrogate mother must be insured against health complications relating to the pregnancy and those arising during her pregnancy.

8. **Will the surrogate mothers like their daughters to do surrogacy?**

The answer to this question by almost all surrogate mothers would be that they would not want their daughters to do surrogacy. But then which option would they choose for their daughters, housemaid, cleaners on the road, bar dancing or sex working. When they answer no to surrogacy, they mean they would like proper employments for their daughters with a career growth. They are doing surrogacy for this very reason, to educate their children and bring better days for them. They are obviously not doing surrogacy for their children to do the same.

9. **Should the surrogate mothers not do employment instead of surrogacy**

   They certainly should if they wish to do so and if this option is available for them. We need to understand the practical problems faced by the uneducated, unskilled poor women who are supportless. If other employment would fulfill their requirements, they would certainly opt for that, but this is easily said than done.

10. **Will the surrogate mother take due care of the baby?**

    It is in her best interest to ensure that the pregnancy goes well. Her objectives are fulfilled when the outcome is good. She has her own children for whom she is doing this. This makes it easy for her to understand the agony of the intended parents. She does care for the baby, but she knows that the baby does not belong to her. It is better for her to consider the arrangement as a contract rather than get emotionally involved. Her mind is better prepared. This may be perceived as not caring for the child. The surrogate mother has experienced those emotions and she is not new to this feeling of motherhood. She is thus capable of handling the emotions that come along.

Glossary

Intended Parent: The parent for whom the surrogate mother will carry the baby for 9 months. They are also called commissioning parents.

Surrogate Mother: The woman who will carry the pregnancy for intended parents and deliver the child.

Gestational Surrogacy: The embryo (pregnancy) is made from the eggs and sperms belonging to the intended parents

Egg Donation Surrogacy: The embryo (pregnancy) is made of eggs borrowed from a different woman and sperms belonging to the intended parents. The borrowing of eggs is sometimes necessary, because the woman's eggs may have finished due to ageing, surgery or disease. This is why women's age is important from fertility point of view. This is not the case with men. Generally, men retain fertility even in their old age.

IUI: Intrauterine insemination: This is a simple treatment in which sperms are released into the womb of a woman for her to achieve a pregnancy. This is done in the woman herself and not the surrogate mother.

IVF/ICSI: Test-tube baby: This is an advanced form of treatment in which the sperms and eggs are put together outside the body(in the laboratory) to create a pregnancy. Normally, this happens in the tubes inside the body of a woman after a sexual relation with a man. This pregnancy is put back into the womb with the help of a fine catheter for it to stick to the womb and grow for nine months.

Embryo: An early stage pregnancy is called an embryo

ICMR: Indian Council for Medical Research: This body was nominated by the government to frame guidelines for the practice of fertility treatment in India.

ART: Assisted Reproductive Technology: If a woman is unable to conceive naturally, she needs to take help of technology. This form of treatment is called Assisted reproduction. In most cases this is done using the eggs and the sperms of the couple, because everyone wants a baby with their own genetic material. If this is not possible for any reason, the pregnancy is done using borrowed eggs or sperms. This involves thorough counseling of the couple. This is only done with full informed consent of the couple.

ART Guidelines: The government nominated the ICMR to develop guidelines to regulate the practice of ART. These guidelines were drafted in 2005 and the newer versions were made in the subsequent years. In 2014, the guidelines were almost ready. As per the guidelines, all ART clinics across India have to be registered. There are set rules and regulations to follow

www.ingramcontent.com/pod-product-compliance
Lightning Source LLC
Chambersburg PA
CBHW020435220526
45464CB00002B/721